The 1(

Mother

U U   U   U   U

Virginia Thorley, OAM, PhD, IBCLC, FILCA
Melissa Clark Vickers, MEd, IBCLC

The 10th Step and Beyond:
Mother Support for Breastfeeding

Editors

Virginia Thorley, OAM, PhD, IBCLC, FILCA

Melissa Clark Vickers, MEd, IBCLC

© Copyright 2012

Hale Publishing, L.P.

1712 N. Forest St.

Amarillo, TX 79106-7017

806-376-9900

800-378-1317

www.iBreastfeeding.com

Library of Congress Control Number: 2012940005

ISBN-13: 978-0-9847746-8-5

Printing and Binding: Edwards Brothers Malloy

Dedication / Acknowledgements

Anything done by anyone on behalf of making the world a better place where breastfeeding works better for mothers and babies is doing a great service. It may seem small, but it all really adds up.

—TED GREINER

This book is dedicated to all who have made the world a better place for breastfeeding mothers and their babies.

There are those who have made our personal world as breastfeeding mothers a better place:

Marian Tompson, who sent me the right breastfeeding advice at the right time, enabling me to begin my breastfeeding journey by reversing an abysmal start.

My children and their families: Nancy and Jeff, Martin and Terri and family, Luke and Andrea and family, and Mary Lise and Don and family.

—VIRGINIA THORLEY

My mother, Juanita Stone Clark, who was my lifelong mothering mentor.

My husband, Bob, for his support and encouragement.

And, of course, my children and their spouses: Dan and Sunny, and Merrilee and Alex, who gave me the reason to experience—and cherish—motherhood.

—MELISSA CLARK VICKERS

Table of Contents

Dedication / Acknowledgements 3

Preface 9

Part I: Mother Support as the 10th Step for
Baby-Friendly Maternity Facilities 11

Introduction Mother Support as Step 10 of the
Baby-Friendly Hospital Initiative 13
Background..13
Why Ten Steps? 13
What Step 10 Means in Practice 15
Definitions 18
The Chapters 18
Conclusion..21

Chapter One Why Breastfeeding Women Need Mother Support 23
Introduction...23
Why Does Breastfeeding Need Special Support?..............................23
What is Mother Support for Breastfeeding? 24
What Does Mother Support Look Like?...25
A Tapestry of Support...32

Chapter Two Mother Support as Part of the Self-Help and
Mutual Aid Movement: Historical Overview..35
Introduction...35
Breastfeeding Groups 37
New Modes of Interaction...39
Group Dynamics and Individual Experience 42
Conclusion...42

Chapter Three Mother Knows Best:La Leche League 45

Part II: Mother Support Around the World: Examples.................................53

Chapter Four Grassroots Mother Support as the Basis for a Large National
Organization: The Australian Breastfeeding Association...............................55
The Australian Breastfeeding Association 59

Chapter Five The Scandinavian Breastfeeding Adventure:
The First Years (1968–78)...63
Personal History...63
The U.S. Sets an Example..63
Unstoppable Scandinavians...64
Mother Support or Mother-To-Mother Support 66

Back to Scandinavia 67

Chapter Six Mother Support in Malaysia **71**
Background...71
Barriers Encountered...73
New Opportunities 73

Chapter Seven Mother Support Group Experience in Paraguay.................**79**
Introduction...79
History of Mother Support in Paraguay 80
Early Link with the Health Professionals 81
Evolution of LLL Support Groups 84
Community Outreach...86
Peer Counselors...89
Baby-Friendly Hospitals 89
Maintaining HCR Mother Support Groups................................92
Problems Faced by Mothers...93
Support From the Community Peer Counselors...........................94
Conclusion..98

**Chapter Eight Peer Counseling for Increasing Exclusive Breastfeeding:
Experiences from Bangladesh** **101**
Introduction...101
Purpose 102
History...102
Monitoring and Evaluation 104
Challenges...108
Conclusions and Scaling Up..109

Chapter Nine The Baby Café **111**
Introduction...111
Purpose and Philosophy 111
History...113
New Opportunities and the Future 116
Barriers..118
Conclusion..118

**Chapter Ten International Organizations and the
Mother-to-Mother Support Group**...**121**

Part III: Moving Forward: Overcoming Barriers to Mother Support...........**131**

**Chapter Eleven Beyond the 10th Step:
The WABA Agenda to Broaden Mother Support Worldwide** **133**
Background...133
History of Mother Support Work in WABA................................134
Global Initiative for Mother Support (GIMS) 137

Implementing the GIMS: MS e-Newsletter, Seed Grant Project, and Others 143
Renewing Global Commitment on Mother Support 145
Today: Where Is the Global Movement on Mother Support? 154
Conclusion 154

Chapter Twelve Supporting Mothers of Infants in the NICU 157
Introduction 157
Rush Mothers' Milk Club (RMMC) 159
Sharing the Science of Human Milk and Lactation 161
Evidence-Based Lactation Technology and Resources 162
Removing Lactation Barriers Specific to Low-Income and African-American
Mothers 163
Integration of BPCs as Primary Lactation Care Providers 164
Breastfeeding Peer Counselors: From Volunteer to a Paid Member of the
NICU Team 164
Mother-to-Mother Support in the Rush Mothers' Milk Club 166
The Shared Experience 167
Peer Counselors and Information, Assistance, and Support 168
"Mothering the Mother" 169
Summary 170

Chapter Thirteen Breastfeeding Support Groups for Mothers of
Multiple-Birth Infants and Children 171
Introduction 171
Birth of a Multiples-Specific Breastfeeding Group 172
It's Complicated 174
Offering Information and Support 176
Postnatal Support 178
Information/Support Group Meeting Logistics 180
Conclusion 182

Chapter Fourteen Overcoming Barriers Through New Technology:
Support Via Text Messaging 183
Introduction 183
Purpose/Philosophy 184
Using SMS in Breastfeeding 185
Developing the MumBubConnect Social Marketing Program 187
Demographics 190
Feeding Behavior 191
Behavioral and Psychological Measures 191
Process Evaluation 192
Lessons Learned 192
Conclusion 193
Acknowledgements 193

Chapter Fifteen Identifying and Overcoming Barriers to the
10th Step in Lalitpur, India 195
Introduction..195
New Commitments...196
Mother Support 196
Evidence...197
The Lalitpur Project..199
Conclusion..202
Acknowledgement 202

Chapter Sixteen Breastfeeding Peer Counselors
in South Africa: Influences of Local Factors....................................203
Introduction..203
Midwife Obstetric Units 204
The Peer Counselor Training Program in Cape Town: Beginnings 204
Male Peer Counselors..205
The Focus Changes...207
Where Are We Now? 208
National Breastfeeding Consultative Meeting......................................208

Chapter Seventeen Sustainability: Why Good Programs Fail and
What We Need to Know 211
Introduction..211
Becoming Known 211
Access to the Support 212
Inclusiveness..213
Financial Sustainability..213
Other Barriers to Sustainability 216
Conclusion..218

Conclusion Going Forth From Here 219

References 223

Index..249

About the Editors...255

Preface

The joy and power of breastfeeding is one of the greatest universal resources.

This natural first food for a newborn life is an amazing and wondrous process that is like a beautiful flower with five petals, each of them representing a vital force of the uniqueness of breastfeeding. It provides irreplaceable immunities and live-saving medicines, total and unbeatable nutrition, while making good economic sense and ecological sense, and, finally, deep love and bonding.

Sadly, this universal and natural culture of breastfeeding, of nurturing the future, was undermined over the last century by those who put profits before health and who manipulated thinking away from the source. Fortunately, the magnificent proliferation of "people power" from all walks of life and from all continents led the United Nations to establish global norms and initiatives to protect, promote, and support breastfeeding. Today, all over the world we are moving back to the great natural gift of breastfeeding, a task with its own great challenges in a fast changing world.

The central figure in the great transformational struggle was the mother, and it is her empowerment and support that was always critical. This book is about supporting the mothers. Virginia Thorley and Melissa Clark Vickers have brought together a truly remarkable mix of 26 people, a team that reflects both the global character of the issue, as well as its multidimensional nature.

The book takes us on a journey that explains not just the historical context and the key concepts, but most importantly the best practices and practical experiences from around the world. It is a journey that addresses both old barriers and new technologies, the continuing practical challenges in moving forward to give life to the culture of breastfeeding, and celebrates the seven real wonders of life—seeing, hearing, touching, tasting, feeding, enjoying, and loving!

We are most grateful to the authors for dedicating the income generated from this book to the work of the World Alliance for Breastfeeding Action (WABA), benefitting not just its core partners, La Leche League International (LLLI), International Baby Food Action Network (IBFAN), International Lactation Consultant Association (ILCA), Wellstart International, and The Academy of Breastfeeding Medicine (ABM), but also the thousands of individuals and institutions that are touched by, and participate in, this galactic network of alliance of alliances through World Breastfeeding Week and its many other enabling activities.

Professor Anwar Fazal, Chairperson Emeritus,

World Alliance for Breastfeeding Action (WABA),

Director, Right Livelihood College, Universiti Sains Malaysia,

Penang, MALAYSIA,

31st December 2011

(Anwar Fazal is a recipient of the Right Livelihood Award, popularly known as the "Alternative Nobel Prize.")

Part 1: Mother Support as the 10th Step for Baby-Friendly Maternity Facilities

Introduction

Mother Support as Step 10 of the Baby-Friendly Hospital Initiative

Virginia Thorley, OAM, PhD, IBCLC, FILCA

Background

When the Baby-Friendly Hospital Initiative (BFHI) was launched in 1991, its basis was the Ten Steps to Successful Breastfeeding, ten best-practice guidelines to provide maternity care that promotes, supports, and protects breastfeeding. The purpose is to give mothers and their babies optimal conditions for a normal start to breastfeeding. The name of this global initiative may be slightly different in some countries, for instance, it is the Mother Baby-Friendly Hospital Initiative (MBFHI) in South Africa, the Baby-Friendly Initiative (BFI) in Britain, and the Baby-Friendly Health Initiative (BFHI) in Australia, but all maternity facilities must reach the global standard for accreditation.

Why Ten Steps?

The concept of Ten Steps came out of the Innocenti Declaration, which was signed by the representatives of 30 countries in Italy in 1990 (Innocenti, 1990; Labbok, 2010). The Ten Steps became the framework on which the Baby-Friendly Hospital Initiative was based when it was launched the following year.

Ten is a round number. We have ten fingers and ten toes, and ten is the basis of our numeral system. The number "10" is often used in lists in religion, philosophy, and popular culture, as it carries a sense of completeness. So it is an apt number for these Steps. There is a further requirement for a hospital or community facility to achieve accreditation as Baby-Friendly: the facility must be compliant with the International Code of Marketing of Breast-Milk Substitutes. The purpose of this Code is to protect mothers from undue influences on their infant-feeding decisions by overt or subtle marketing by commercial entities. Such influences had long been highly effective marketing tools for products associated with the artificial feeding of infants, through drawing mothers away from breastfeeding their babies. As noted by the late Dr. Wah Wong, the requirement for maternity facilities to comply with the International Code is a virtual eleventh step, but the number of Ten Steps has been maintained.

The Ten Steps

The Ten Steps to Successful Breastfeeding are set out in Figure I.1.

Figure I.1. The Ten Steps to Successful Breastfeeding

1. Have a written breastfeeding policy that is routinely communicated to all healthcare staff.
2. Train all healthcare staff in skills necessary to implement this policy.
3. Inform all pregnant women about the benefits and management of breastfeeding.
4. Place babies in skin-to-skin contact with their mothers immediately following birth for at least an hour and encourage mothers to recognize when their babies are ready to breastfeed, offering help if needed.
5. Show mothers how to breastfeed and how to maintain lactation, even if they should be separated from their infants.
6. Give newborn infants no food or drink other than breastmilk, unless medically indicated.
7. Practice rooming-in, allow mothers and infants to remain together-24 hours a day.
8. Encourage breastfeeding on demand.
9. Give no artificial teats or dummies to breastfeeding infants.
10. Foster the establishment of breastfeeding support and refer mothers on discharge from the facility.

Step 1 requires the facility to have a written breastfeeding policy. This policy must cover all of the 10 Steps and specifically address implementation of each Step. Furthermore, the policy must be readily accessible, with summaries posted in all areas where pregnant women, mothers, and children are likely to be. (An example would be rooms for changing babies' diapers, anywhere in the facility.) What is more, the summary of the breastfeeding policy must be in the relevant community languages. Steps 2 and 3 cover education for staff and pregnant women. Steps 4 to 9 cover maternity care that supports the mother and baby to begin their breastfeeding relationship and avoid iatrogenic (staff-caused) problems from developing (WHO/UNICEF, 2009).

Step 10, the subject of this book, is designed to ensure that the mother and her baby do not return to the community unsupported. A birthing facility is mandated to provide contact details for support after the mother leaves the hospital, so she does not lose confidence in her ability to nourish her baby from her own body, is supported to recognize her baby's hunger cues and how to position and attach her baby so that both are comfortable and the baby is drinking, and knows when to seek help. Support is also needed in an environment in which substitutes for her milk, and equipment to put it in, are promoted to her by the people around her and through advertising—and that means in much of the world. Support can be informal, such as from family members or the shopkeeper who finds her a chair so she can breastfeed when her baby needs to. More formal support is the subject of many of the chapters that follow.

What Step 10 Means in Practice

The chapters that follow address the various forms that mother support has taken in a variety of settings. Some of the authors address specific groups or programs. Others discuss the question of mother support more broadly, providing a context for it and conceptualizing it, to give the reader a comprehensive guide for implementing support for mothers that is timely and appropriate to the mothers and to the setting in which they find themselves. After all, what mothers need is the *right support* from the *right person* at the *right time*. Some of the programs or groups described are based on volunteers and were established by mothers in the community, who continue to provide the leadership. They provide mother-to-mother support; that is, support for mothers by other mothers, and often they provide other forms of support, too. Two of these chapters, one by Elisabet Helsing and one by Karen Kerkhoff Gromada, are written as personal accounts to provide insights into how a need was identified and how mothers found ways to provide the appropriate support. Many of the groups described in this book provide mother support from unpaid, volunteer breastfeeding counselors (BFCs), with some degree of training by the organization. Thus, they are women who can afford to provide volunteer hours. Some programs provide mother-to-mother support from breastfeeding peer counselors (BPCs or PCs); that is, women with breastfeeding experience from the local, often poor communities. These women often find they cannot volunteer their time without a small stipend. Without it, they would need to take other paid work and be lost to the program. This means that funding is essential to maintain the program.

Other programs described in this book are organized by health professionals, and involve both peer counselors and paid workers. These programs include the Lalitpur Project in Uttar Pradesh, India.

The authors show a degree of diversity, based on background and experience, as to their preference for mother-controlled support initiatives, such as mother-to-mother support groups, peer-counselor programs led by professionals, such as in the highly specialized area of the Neonatal Intensive Care Unit (NICU), or a blend of models. In truth, there is good evidence to support a blend of lay and professional support to provide optimal support to the breastfeeding mother (Britton et al., 2007). A longer chapter, by Sarah Amin, Rebecca Magalhães, and Paulina Smith, describes how the World Alliance for Breastfeeding Action (WABA) has taken the question of support for mothers to breastfeed beyond the usual interpretation of the 10th Step of the BFHI to involve the community in ways that were not envisaged when the 10 Steps were first described in the Innocenti Declaration (1990). Indeed, this chapter opens up many ways in which mothers can be supported to breastfeed after they leave the hospital, measures which may be new to readers of this book.

As can be expected, both lay breastfeeding counselors and breastfeeding peer counselors are usually women. However, in some situations, one or more men have become involved, undergoing the same training as their female colleagues. The men undertake many of the same responsibilities as the women, depending on the cultural environment as regards what is considered appropriate. They are a particular asset in speaking man-to-man with fathers, providing information that is consistent with what the other lay breastfeeding counselors provide. Examples in this book of the use of male BPCs include the Rush Mothers' Milk Club (RMMC) in a Neonatal Intensive Care unit (NICU) in Chicago, which until recently had one male BPC, communities which had some male BPCs in Western Cape, South Africa, and in Paraguay, where two men undertook peer counselor training in an organization called "Parhupar." Being a "peer," for both women and men, is defined by the program. It may mean being part of the community, as in Western Cape and Paraguay, or being the mother of twins, triplets, and other multiples in special groups for mothers of multiples. In the case of the RMMC, "peer" means having experienced being the parent of a baby in the NICU. The role of a male BPC in the special environment of a NICU is described thus:

> The RMMC BPC program is unique in that it has employed a male BPC. The BPC role for a male is slightly different from the female role. As a male BPC, Henry does not directly assist

mothers with pumping and breastfeeding. He does, however, carry out all other aspects of the NICU BPC role. Henry demonstrates for families how to keep pump equipment clean during and after milk collection; he assists with the breast pump rental program; he shares lactation related research articles and handouts with families; he attends and contributes to the weekly Mother's Milk Club meetings; he performs twice daily milk checks throughout the unit; he greets visiting parents and is a source of support and encouragement for families; he provides any needed lactation supplies; he answers questions and reviews teaching of milk collection, transport, and storage; and he meets with mothers in the ante partum unit to discuss the benefits of providing mother's milk. Henry reaches out to fathers in the NICU and is able to connect with them on a uniquely personal yet professional level. As a father who has seen first-hand the benefits of human milk for his own child, Henry enjoys sharing the "before and after" photos of Miracle: first as a tiny one-pound preemie in the NICU, and now as a thriving and healthy child. He delivers his own powerful and personal message that mother's milk made a difference for Miracle, which is a source of hope and empowerment for the current NICU families when they need it most (Beverly Rossman, personal communication, December 2011).

Implementation of Step 10 also requires maternity facilities to establish effective referral to mother support in the community as part of their discharge planning for new mothers. It is not enough to provide a leaflet with the contact details of a local form of breastfeeding support and believe that this is all that is needed. Maternity facilities need to:

- Provide contact details of all suitable breastfeeding support options in the local area where the individual mother lives.

- Ensure that she has access to appropriate breastfeeding support 24/7.

- Ensure that the contact details are up-to-date.

The maternity facility that establishes contact with mother support groups and encourages contact between the leaders of the groups in the antenatal clinic or postnatal wards can establish a seamless transition to community support as the mother has already met women from these groups and the facility's endorsement of such support is obvious. Similarly, the hospital or clinic that links mothers into a peer counselor program, a drop-in center run by health workers, or a blend of volunteers or health workers is making sure the mother has access to the support she needs. The chapters that follow describe programs and movements, which add to the possibilities.

Local culture also plays a part in how the support is provided in special circumstances. For instance, for tiny babies in the NICU who are as yet unable to go directly to the breast or are in the process of transitioning to the breast, in many parts of the world, the most viable means of providing their mothers' milk is by expressing the milk manually, that is, hand expression. This method is affordable and can be done in the absence of electrical power, such as during storms and natural disasters, and in village settings (Thorley, 2011a). For instance, in chapter 9 Pushpa Panadam mentions how mothers of babies in the NICU in Paraguay are encouraged and supported to hand express their milk. In Chicago in the United States, the emphasis by staff and peer counselors is on providing mechanical assistance, in the form of breast pumps, to mothers of babies in the NICU, who are supported by the Rush Mothers' Milk Club (chapter 12). Mothers in New Zealand are taught hand-expression of their milk as part of the BFHI, but when milk expression for many months is necessary, they are counseled about the use of hospital-grade pumps (chapter 17). The most suitable means of expressing milk appears to depend on the individual circumstances, rather than the method used (Becker, Cooney, & Smith, 2011).

Definitions

Each chapter defines its use of terms, but across the book, "mother support" encompasses many modes of support of the new mother to breastfeed her baby or babies. It includes the mother-to-mother support of the mother-led breastfeeding groups that arose from the 1950s onwards and peer counselor programs, which evolved later. Some chapter authors have abbreviated "mother-to-mother support" to "MtMS." "Mother support" includes programs initiated by the hospitals themselves, whether antenatal or postnatal, and support given within the hospital by volunteers from mother support groups who are welcomed into the hospital. As Chapter 11 points out, it includes a much greater range of informal support from others in the community, such as men, youth, family, and others.

The Chapters

In chapter 1, Melissa Vickers provides the very important explanation of why breastfeeding mothers need support, thus establishing the need for support. This provides the context and rationale for the chapters that discuss provision of that support, which comprise the rest of the book. In chapter 2, Virginia Thorley places mother support groups in the context of the self-help and mutual support movement. As well as demonstrating that these groups fit the characteristics of a self-help group, the author traces the development of modes of self-help beyond the earlier concept of the face-to-face mode as the means of mutual support, through the rise of new technologies. This broadening of how individuals seek and use groups for the support they need applies as much to breastfeeding groups as to the broader self-help movement. Section I concludes with the chapter by Kaye Lowman Boorom in which she describes the formation and early growth of La Leche League, the pioneering group which influenced the development of mother-to-mother support for breastfeeding women around the world. Founded in Chicago in 1956, La Leche League led the way in showing that the volunteer efforts of mothers could not only make a difference in breastfeeding for individual mothers, but also influence the health professions, institutions, and government policies.

The seven chapters in Part II provide examples of mother support around the world. Chapters 4 to 7 describe groups in a number of countries. In chapter 4, Nina Berry sets the large Australian organization, the Australian Breastfeeding Association (formerly the Nursing Mothers' Association of Australia) within the context of grassroots mother support, as well as political advocacy. In chapter 5, Elisabet Helsing, the founder of the Norwegian organization, Ammehjelpen, describes the formation of the Scandinavian groups, each adapted to the milieu of the particular country—Norway, Sweden, and Denmark. Siti Norjinah Moin, in chapter 6, provides information about the formation and growth of the Malaysian mother support group, *Persatuan Penasihat Penyusuan Ibu Malaysia* (PPPIM). She describes the challenges faced when the expatriates who had helped form the PPPIM groups left the country, and the difficulty of finding enough volunteer hours since most local women work. The organization took up new opportunities, linking with other local organizations on shared issues, eventually becoming involved in global networks. Chapter 7, by Pushpa Panadam, provides a case study of the establishment of mother support groups in Paraguay. This begins with the work of La Leche League of Paraguay (LLLPy), whose groups attract mainly better educated, urban women, and includes their collaboration with healthcare professionals and LLLPy's outreach work in hospitals and in disadvantaged sections of the community. This long chapter goes on to describe the work of peer counselors, who support poorer women in their local communities, including in the hospitals. The chapter also discusses the ramifications of Paraguay's bi-lingual status in relation to supporting breastfeeding mothers and pregnant women, and other challenges.

Chapter 8 turns from mother support groups to peer counseling. Rukhsana Haider describes the effectiveness of a peer counselor program in Bangladesh in a poor urban area and a rural area. The innovative Baby Café concept developed in England, and now spreading to the United States, New Zealand, and other countries, is the subject of chapter 9, by Catherine Pardoe and Julie Williams. The concept of drop-in centers to support and encourage breastfeeding mothers has been tried before, but financial sustainability has been a barrier for many programs in different regions. The authors describe how the concept of a brand is working for Baby Café. Maryanne Stone-Jimenez and Judiann McNulty have contributed a chapter on international programs. Using examples from a number of settings to provide insights into effective programs, their chapter fittingly concludes Section II. This chapter emphasizes the value of storytelling in mother-to-mother support groups—whether the focus is on exclusive breastfeeding in the first six months or on continued breastfeeding after appropriate, locally available complementary foods are introduced at about six months.

The seven chapters in Part III, Overcoming Barriers to Mother Support, present a diverse range of situations. Titled "Beyond the 10th Step," the lead chapter for this section, by Sarah Amin, Rebecca Magalhães, and Paulina Smith, presents an expansion of the idea of mother support beyond the basic concept set out in the wording of Step 10 of the "Ten Steps to Successful Breastfeeding." This long chapter presents a wealth of diverse modes of providing the mother with the support she needs. The authors explore mothers' needs today and describe how the World Alliance for Breastfeeding Action (WABA) has broadened the application of mother support beyond the concept of the mother-to-mother support group to a whole raft of support involving the community. Mother-to-mother support, they argue, is still a part of the picture, but it is not the whole picture; instead, it is part of a rich tapestry of other modes.

Other chapters in Section III also discuss newer modes of provision of mother support to meet new needs or to meet old needs in a different way. In chapter 12, Beverly Rossman and colleagues describe the special situation of supporting the mothers of tiny babies in the Neonatal Intensive Care Unit (NICU) at Rush Mothers' Milk Club in Chicago to provide mother's own milk. Many of the mothers belong to sections of the community where breastfeeding is unusual, even for babies born at term. The authors describe the challenges such a program has to overcome on a daily basis, including uncertainty about the baby's condition and the prospect of expressing their milk for a considerable period. They present the example of how an innovative program in the NICU, the Rush Mothers' Milk Club, has created impressive rates of breastmilk feeding in the unit.

Mothers of twins, triplets, and other multiples face the problems of prematurity more often than in the general population, and they have more than one baby to contend with. After the birth of her twins, Karen Kerkhoff Gromada saw the need for specific, targeted support for mothers of multiples, which the regular breastfeeding groups can only do to some extent. In Chapter 13, she describes the formation of specific groups within LLL to support mothers of multiples.

Many new mothers today belong to the generation that uses the new electronic technology for information and support, and prefer to turn to hand-held mobile devices and social media sites for information and support, rather than to traditional face-to-face groups. In chapter 14, Rebekah Russell-Bennett and her colleagues in Brisbane, Queensland, Australia, describe an innovative program that uses text messaging, on demand, to provide support when the mothers need it. Komal Kushwaha, in chapter 15, describes the barriers to implementing Step 10 in Uttar Pradesh, India, and how the Lalitpur Project addresses these barriers. This project uses several levels of lay and professional workers to ensure that the new mother has support in her own village to enable her to practice exclusive breastfeeding and to introduce appropriate, locally available complementary foods at about the age of six months.

In Chapter 16, Jean Ridler and Rosemary Gauld discuss the beginnings and eventual decline of breastfeeding peer counseling in Western Cape, South Africa, including the emergence of a few males as peer counselors supporting breastfeeding. They, too, describe the use of storytelling in the cultural context. This chapter also provides insights into why excellent programs are not sustained, particularly when funding is reallocated elsewhere. Virginia Thorley's chapter on "Sustainability" discusses why good programs fail and what we need to know to address these issues. The examples used in this chapter include some from the preceding chapters, while also introducing new examples. A short concluding chapter rounds off the book.

CONCLUSION

The editors hope that this text will provide materials and discussion points for a diverse range of individuals and organizations concerned with the provision of mother support, so mothers will be encouraged in breastfeeding their babies. The target audience for this book includes hospitals and health centers; state and national Departments of Health; non-government organizations (NGOs); United Nations bodies; Baby-Friendly Hospital Committees at institutional, state, and national levels; and individuals.

Without support in the community, the existing situation will continue, where relatively few mother-baby dyads reach the internationally recommended six months of exclusive, unsupplemented breastfeeding, followed by the continuation of breastfeeding after the introduction of appropriate complementary foods (WHO/UNICEF, 2003). The goal of all of us is that the mother will be provided with the *right support* from the *right person* at the *right time*.

Chapter One

Why Breastfeeding Women Need Mother Support

Melissa Clark Vickers, MEd, IBCLC

INTRODUCTION

Mother Support for breastfeeding: the topic is both obvious and elusive, and has changed over time. Centuries ago, no one spoke of the need for mother support, no one researched how to do it, no one gave a lot of thought to it; it was a given. Women looked to other women—their friends and family—for help in raising their children. In eras when breastfeeding was valued and practiced, women learned the art of breastfeeding effortlessly through observation, and it was assumed that a newborn would be nourished at his mother's breast. Those babies, who, for whatever reason including fashion, did not breastfeed, were likely doomed to illness and death.

> The need for mother support has not changed over the millennia; but the need to talk about it, document it, research it, and fund it, has. With the destruction of traditional systems of support, new ones need to be established and strengthened. (Vickers, 2009)

WHY DOES BREASTFEEDING NEED SPECIAL SUPPORT?

Breastfeeding is something very personal. If a baby cannot attach to the breast or refuses to eat, the mother may feel that as personal rejection or that her baby "doesn't like" her breast. If her baby is not growing well, perhaps because she has been influenced by advice to make her baby wait for feeds, thus limiting the stimulation to her milk supply, the mother feels she is personally failing her baby. The bottle-feeding mother is likely to see refusal of a feed in a different light, accepting that her baby is simply not hungry. If her baby has difficulty drinking from the bottle, she is likely to change the brand of bottle or nipple, sometimes several times—but she will not take it as a personal judgment by her baby.

Any of these reasons—unsuccessful attempts to latch a hungry baby, refusal of the breast, or poor weight gains—typically undermine a mother's confidence in her ability to breastfeed. Yet, stress and lack of confidence can interfere with the ability of her breasts to "let down" and eject the milk that is there, so her baby can access it. Derrick B. Jelliffe and E.F.P. Jelliffe (1978) wrote: "Lactation has been termed a 'confidence trick,' and failure in healthy well-nourished women with normal full-term babies is more frequently due to the 'anxiety-nursing-failure cycle,' based on emotional interference with the let-down reflex." Believing is achieving. This is where mother support is a valuable aid. An important facet of what the experienced mother, the peer counselor, or the healthcare worker do when providing one-on-one support is reassuring the mother and building her confidence. Even better, if they encourage more skin-to-skin contact between mother and baby, the oxytocin levels in both will rise. Oxytocin aids bonding, but it also triggers the milk ejection reflex (MER) that causes the milk to "let down" (Lawrence & Lawrence, 2011, pp. 258-260).

What is Mother Support for Breastfeeding?

Mother support is simple and timeless, yet elusive. When it is present and working as it should, it is such a natural process that trying to define it seems as unnecessary as defining breathing. When it is absent or weak, we are more likely to look at the problems that result than to address head-on the role that adequate support might have played in preventing those problems.

In its broadest terms, Mother Support is "any support provided to mothers for the purpose of improving breastfeeding practices of both mother and infant/young child" (WABA, 2007b). This definition is broad because Mother Support comes in many forms and serves many purposes. It includes the gentle encouragement and guidance that the grandmother gives her daughter with a new baby, as well as government regulations put in place to say officially, "You may not prevent this mother from breastfeeding." It covers the healthcare providers who work with the mother whose baby is unable to breastfeed effectively, as well as the lay breastfeeding counselors who help mothers learn the art of breastfeeding by modeling and encouragement.

Who Needs It?

Often, we think of "support" as something given to someone in dire need—financial support for the poor, mental health support for the emotionally unstable, life support for the critically ill. Certainly support is important in these situations, and in the context of breastfeeding, support is critical to breastfeeding success in times of crisis or situations such as these:

- The mother who is having difficulty getting her newborn to latch on to her breast comfortably and efficiently.
- The mother of the tiny preterm infant born too early.
- The mother and baby coping in the midst of a natural disaster—flood, hurricane/cyclone, earthquake.
- The mother whose illness requires treatment or medication that could be harmful to her breastfeeding infant.
- The mother who has been asked to leave a public place because she is breastfeeding her infant.
- The mother whose confidence in her body's ability to nourish her baby is undermined by negative comments or conflicting advice.

Equally important—arguably more important—is the kind of broad-based support that creates the breastfeeding culture in which it is both the cultural and biological norm. It is the seamless kind of support that makes breastfeeding as natural as breathing:

- The new mother who is eager to learn how to care for her newborn.
- The mother who just needs a little reassurance that breastfeeding is going well.
- The mother who is returning to work and wants to continue to breastfeed her infant.
- The mother who is discovering the joys of breastfeeding her toddler.
- The mother who wants to share her breastfeeding experience with other mothers.

So Mother Support for Breastfeeding is a blend of encouragement, problem solving, normalizing, and protection.

WHAT DOES MOTHER SUPPORT LOOK LIKE?

Mother Support for Breastfeeding can be as subtle as a knowing smile from one woman to another woman breastfeeding her infant. It can be as obvious as the healthcare provider giving hands-on assistance for a specific breastfeeding problem or the legislature passing the law that protects mothers breastfeeding in public places.

In 2008, the World Alliance for Breastfeeding Action (WABA) chose Mother Support for Breastfeeding as its theme for World Breastfeeding

Week (WBW): "Mother Support: Going for the Gold." Taking advantage of the 2008 Olympics happening the same month (August), the Action Folder chose the symbolism of the five Olympic logo rings to represent various arenas of support for breastfeeding. Rather than the more linear arrangement in the Olympic logo, the Folder recognizes the interconnection and overlapping of the five types of support, as well as the critical role that women themselves play in each of the five types—both as women needing the support and as women giving the support. Thus it conceptualizes the five interlocking rings surrounding and overlapping with the center circle— women (Figure 1.1).

Figure 1.1. WABA Circles

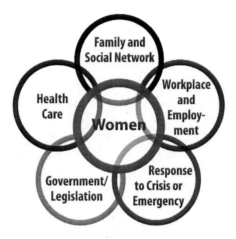

Circle: Women in the Center

Women not only receive support from many sources, they actively secure support and provide it as well. Women are key players in all CIRCLES. Strong support in the outer circle creates a growing power in the center that radiates out to the other circles of support. The strong network of mother-to-mother support organizations around the world, founded and maintained by women, are a vital demonstration of this concept.

Over the course of history, women learned the value of networking with other women: learning new skills, sharing good times, leaning on each other in challenging times. In traditional settings, the network consisted of extended family members—mothers, grandmothers, sisters, and aunts— who were close by and readily accessible (WABA, 2008).

The role of women has broadened considerably and encompasses much more than home and family. Expanded roles strengthen the need for networking. Sadly, many women today do not have a network of support to call upon. Extended family members are not always geographically close, so women rely on non-family members and, when available, on technological innovations, such as the telephone and Internet. When all the Circles are strong and provide seamless mother support for breastfeeding, the result is truly empowering for future generations.

The goal is that in whatever direction in the center circle a mother turns, she receives positive and empathetic support for her breastfeeding experience.

Circle: Family and Social Network

This Circle represents what women have been doing for millennia: seeking and offering support in a very personal way. Women, by their very nature, are nurturing and thrive in a shared community of women with similar interests, problems, and circumstances. They are comfortable moving in and out of the position of needing support—one day a mother will seek support, and the next will offer support. The wisdom of women is a collective experience that builds on the successes and failures of others, and recognizes the need for tailoring the information to fit the needs of the individual woman and her family.

Women depend on support from the family, and this is especially true for breastfeeding support. Family members—spouses/partners, parents, siblings, and extended family—who fully support a mother's breastfeeding play an important role in her success. "Full support" implies at least a minimal knowledge base about breastfeeding, an understanding of why it is important, and the basics of how it works. With that kind of knowledge, family supporters can be both cheerleaders and co-problem-solvers.

Often, family members will understand the value of breastfeeding, but have little direct knowledge of how breastfeeding works. This is especially true in cultures where bottle-feeding is the norm. In this situation, the family member can be an effective cheerleader, but may interfere with appropriate problem solving, even with the best of intentions. Yet, sometimes family members *don't* value breastfeeding, *don't* understand it, and *don't* support it. This makes it challenging for the mother who wants to breastfeed, but needs at least some encouragement or a place to turn for questions.

These three categories of family support—supportive/knowledgeable, supportive/not knowledgeable, and not supportive—reflect the kind of support a woman may find within her social network of friends and co-workers, who can make up for lack of family support, or make that lack even more insurmountable.

The social network extends to the media as well. The information that a woman finds about breastfeeding from media she trusts, be it magazines, books, Internet, or social media, can reinforce her breastfeeding experience or seriously undermine it.

It is clear that an integral part of providing Mother Support for Breastfeeding is ensuring that the people breastfeeding mothers come in contact with are also supportive and knowledgeable. This is no small task!

Circle: Healthcare

Just as birth has become increasingly medicalized, so, too, has breastfeeding. For the many women who give birth in a hospital, it is often the healthcare provider who provides the initial support for those first breastfeeds. Just as family members may be knowledgeable and/or supportive of breastfeeding, healthcare providers can be a wonderful source of support and encouragement—or a major impediment. Because the healthcare provider is often seen as the official expert, it makes the need for knowledgeable and supportive healthcare providers all the more important.

Fortunately, the Baby-Friendly Hospital Initiative (BFHI) has provided the means to document and encourage support and training for breastfeeding support, at least in the hospital setting. Because becoming "Baby-Friendly" is done by choice and not mandated, however, the need is still great for ensuring support from healthcare providers.

It is important to note that this need does not only apply to those healthcare providers who routinely work in the labor/delivery/postpartum hospital or clinic areas. It also applies to *any* healthcare provider the breastfeeding mother may turn to for medical help. The dermatologist the mother consults with for a rash, or the pediatrician she brings her sick child to, or the breast surgeon she consults about a suspicious lump all need to understand the reasons for protecting breastfeeding as much possible and how to go about doing that.

Circle: Government and Legislation

Government policy and legislation are essential in supporting women in many aspects of their lives. Governments have the authority to make laws, to adjudicate disputes, and to issue administrative decisions. Laws and public policies are needed to support a breastfeeding mother. When governments implement the International Code of Marketing of Breast-Milk Substitutes and subsequent World Health Assembly resolutions, mothers are protected from commercial influences that undermine breastfeeding success (WABA, 2008).

When societal pressures alone are not strong enough to support the breastfeeding woman and her baby, government regulations can provide support—albeit artificially imposed—to ensure that breastfeeding is not interfered with. In the United States, while there are no federal breastfeeding policies *per se*, most states have enacted some form of breastfeeding legislation to support a woman's right to breastfeed her baby. None of the states have (or ever had) laws *prohibiting* breastfeeding, so the point of the legislation has been to make it clear that breastfeeding *is* legal. Most states have done little more than pass laws stating a woman's right to breastfeed anywhere she and her baby can legally be, yet few have any kind of punishment clause for those who would interfere.

The judicial branch of government is often involved in settling civil disputes with the potential for interfering with breastfeeding. Judges—who may or may not be knowledgeable or supportive—may be the decision-makers for divorce cases in which the father's desire for custody and/or visitation would necessarily disrupt or even terminate any breastfeeding. When parents are willing to work in the best interests of the child—which include not only continuing the breastfeeding relationship, but the relationship between the father and child—a settlement can be reached that allows for generous, but shorter visitation periods until the child is old enough for longer separations.

Sometimes government support comes not in the form of official laws and policies, but instead in the form of documents that make both the reasons to breastfeed and the need for support clear. A recent United States example of this is the *Surgeon General's Call to Action to Support Breastfeeding* (USDHHS, 2011). The Call to Action included 20 recommended actions for individuals, healthcare officials, and governments to take to support and encourage breastfeeding, starting with #1: "Give mothers support they need" (Table 1.1). Each action is followed by a series of recommended implementation strategies to achieve the action. While this is not legislation, it does effectively say that breastfeeding is important and worth protecting, promoting, and supporting.

Table 1.1. The U.S. *Surgeon General's Call to Action for Breastfeeding:* 20 Recommended Actions.

1. Give mothers the support they need.

2. Develop programs to educate fathers and grandmothers about breastfeeding.

3. Strengthen programs that provide mother-to-mother support and peer counseling.

4. Use community-based organizations to promote and support breastfeeding.

5. Create a national campaign to promote breastfeeding.

6. Ensure that the marketing of infant formula is conducted in a way that minimizes its negative impacts on exclusive breastfeeding.

7. Ensure that maternity care practices throughout the United States are fully supportive of breastfeeding.

8. Develop systems to guarantee continuity of skilled support for lactation between hospitals and healthcare settings in the community.

9. Provide education and training in breastfeeding for all health professionals who care for women and children.

10. Include basic support for breastfeeding as a standard of care for midwives, obstetricians, family physicians, nurse practitioners, and pediatricians.

11. Ensure access to services provided by International Board Certified Lactation Consultants.

12. Identify and address obstacles to greater availability of safe banked donor milk for fragile infants.

13. Work toward establishing paid maternity leave for all employed mothers.

14. Ensure that employers establish and maintain comprehensive, high-quality lactation support programs for their employees.

15. Expand the use of programs in the workplace that allow lactating mothers to have direct access to their babies.

16. Ensure that all childcare providers accommodate the needs of breastfeeding mothers and infants.

17. Increase funding of high-quality research on breastfeeding.

18. Strengthen existing capacity and develop future capacity for conducting research on breastfeeding.

19. Develop a national monitoring system to improve the tracking of breastfeeding rates, as well as the policies and environmental factors that affect breastfeeding.

20. Improve national leadership on the promotion and support of breastfeeding.

Included in these Actions (#19) is the recommendation for a national monitoring system to track breastfeeding rates. The U.S. Centers for Disease Control and Prevention publishes a yearly "Breastfeeding Report Card" that provides a state-by-state progress report on various factors indicative of breastfeeding rates (CDC, 2011). And improving breastfeeding rates—initiation, exclusivity, and duration—is a part of the United States national Healthy People 2020 Goals recently released (HealthyPeople.gov, 2011).

Circle: Workplace and Employment

Every woman is a working woman. Some, out of choice or necessity, work outside of the home and are temporarily away from their breastfeeding infants. Workplace policies that allow for on-site daycare (including having the breastfeeding infant with his mother as she works), mandated breaks to allow her to breastfeed or express her milk, and lactation support for employees increase the likelihood that a mother will continue to at least provide her milk for her infant, indirectly if not directly.

As early as 1919, breastfeeding breaks in the workplace were being recommended. The International Labor Organization (ILO) Maternity Protection Convention of 1919 recommended that breastfeeding mothers should be allowed two 30-minute breaks during work hours to breastfeed their babies (ILO, 1919). Recent healthcare reform in the U.S. included a "Break Time for Nursing Mothers"[1] law (US Department of Labor, 2010) in the Patient Protection and Affordable Care Act (PPACA) passed last year. This is a first step to ensuring that breastfeeding mothers have time and a place to pump or express milk during their work day.

---

1   Note that in the United States, "nursing" is synonymous with "breastfeeding," (in addition to the medical usage). In other parts of the world, "nursing" refers more to the act of providing care, but not necessarily breastfeeding.

Another avenue of support for the working mother comes before the need for nursing breaks—that is, adequate maternity leave that allows for a longer period of protected time off from work after a baby is born. The longer a mother can stay home with her baby to get breastfeeding well-established and to let her body fully recover from pregnancy and delivery, the better the chances of a longer breastfeeding experience. Some countries provide better maternity leave policies than others.

Circle: Response to Crisis or Emergency

Crisis or emergency can put the Mother Support for Breastfeeding to the real test. From the WABA 2008 Action Folder:

> When a mother finds herself under stress due to events outside her control, her responsibility to her children elevates from one of nurturing to one of survival. She may need to find safe housing, food, and clothing, while also struggling to communicate with other family members, support agencies, and healthcare workers.

> During natural disasters or in areas affected by war or conflict, families are uprooted from their homes and communities, and find themselves in unfamiliar places. Social agencies that care for children and families can support the breastfeeding mother by providing items that every mother needs: sufficient food, water, and clothing. A mother's milk may be the only safe food available for her baby under these circumstances.

Recommendations for those who support breastfeeding mothers in these emergencies are available—see the Emergency Nutrition Network for examples (www.ennonline.net). Crisis situations are not limited to natural disasters. Health crises for either mother or baby require additional support to be in place to manage and maintain breastfeeding when possible.

A TAPESTRY OF SUPPORT

When mothers are adequately supported to breastfeed, everyone—the baby, the mother, the family, the community—benefits. This kind of support, coming from many different facets of society, helps move us toward breastfeeding as the cultural norm and weaves a tapestry of support. Tapestries are both beautiful and strong, and the beauty and strength come from the diversity of types of support interwoven together. While any form of support can help a mother breastfeed her child, the synergistic effect of the tapestry makes it easier on that mother, empowering her to support other mothers. Ted Greiner has stated this idea succinctly:

> Anything done by anyone on behalf of making the world a better place where breastfeeding works better for mothers and babies is doing a great service. It may seem small, but it all really adds up (WABA, 2008).

Chapter Two

Mother Support as Part of the Self-Help and Mutual Aid Movement: Historical Overview

Virginia Thorley, OAM, PhD, IBCLC, FILCA

INTRODUCTION

Members of mother support groups seldom view themselves in the wider context of the self-help movement, whereby groups of citizens come together to provide mutual support to supplement what is provided by other individuals and services. Yet breastfeeding groups established for mothers to support each other and the new mothers in the community are a form of self-help group. Those involved in mother support groups can learn from the wider context of self-help. This chapter will discuss groups that provide support to breastfeeding mothers within the context of the self-help and mutual aid genre. New technology is creating even wider communities of people who would never otherwise meet, and mutually supportive interactions are part of this. My metaphor for the self-help, mutual aid, and self-care movement is a galaxy, rather than a single planet or even one solar system. Within the many diverse groups providing various forms of support in this imaginary galaxy, mother support is like a sun with many planets.

Defining Self-Help

The original model of self-help and mutual support was the extended family and kinship system. Extended families (kin) and networks of neighbors and friends (kith) provided a safety net, and even today, where family networks have broken down, isolated individuals sometimes form informal family-like groups (Caplan, 1990). Long before the growth of cities, clans and tribes needed cooperation and mutual assistance to survive. Later, religious institutions of many faiths provided mutual assistance to support their members, and sometimes the stranger or traveler, also. After feudalism disintegrated in Europe, craft guilds and unions provided support for their peers, and this sometimes included activism (Katz & Bender, 1990, pp. 9-21). During this time, the Freemasons expanded well beyond its origins as a craft guild to support its members in difficult times (Caplan, 1990). In the 250 years to 1800 came the growth of "friendly societies," originally based on occupational groups, which provided assistance to their members in sickness or hard times (Katz & Bender, 1990). Because these groups also campaigned for better social or workplace conditions for their members, they sometimes faced opposition from the powerbrokers in their societies. Indeed, in the 1830s when a group of farm laborers in Dorset, England, formed a friendly society to protest against declining wages, these "Tolpuddle Martyrs," as they were later called, were transported to Australia as convicts. Many of today's self-help groups, including the breastfeeding groups, are involved in some degree of activism for the benefits of those they assist (Thorley, 2011b).

Alfred H. Katz believed that the dislocation felt by many individuals in industrialized societies helped to explain the growth of self-help groups (Katz, 2003-2004). The shrinking of the family to the nuclear family, without the immediate support of a wider network of kith and kin, has created new pressures, as there are fewer individuals to share the load (Caplan, 1990). So support from experts or from various groups of peers has come to fill the gap. Self-help groups of many sorts grew in numbers in the second half of the 20th century, encompassing small and large groups, from those struggling to become known to national or even international associations. In some countries "clearinghouses" were begun to assist small groups with few resources and provide referrals, as well as providing advice on how to begin a group. Surveys in the late-1980s found that concerns felt by groups were predominantly related to survival; that is, finding members and becoming known (Wituk, Ealey, Brown, Shepherd, & Meissen, 2005). Fifteen years later Scott Wituk and colleagues from the Self-Help Network, a clearinghouse for self-help groups in Kansas, USA, surveyed a random sample of 250 groups from the 1,500 Kansas groups they identified as meeting their criteria. That is, they were comprised of members with a common situation; their main mode was "mutual assistance"; and they had a minimum of one telephone contact number (Wituk et al., 2005). By then, shorter hospital stays and changes in healthcare funding had impacted how individuals sought health advice and created challenges for groups. Mutual support and useful information were considered the primary benefits of group membership. As in the earlier surveys, becoming known and recruitment to the group were the major concerns identified (Wituk et al., 2005). These findings were seen as endorsing the need for self-help clearinghouses to put individuals in need of specific support and small support groups in touch with each other (Wituk et al., 2005).

Other modern manifestations of the self-help group include those organized for the poorest members of society, such as the local groups formed to provide micro credit in Tamil Nadu, India. Unlike self-help groups formed by individuals themselves, they have official involvement in how the groups are managed. These groups involve individuals who contribute to a common fund, the money being loaned to support businesses, such as craft occupations, to encourage self-sustainability (Directorate of Town Panchayats, 2010). Although the focus of breastfeeding groups is on mother-to-mother support of a health-enhancing activity, financial sustainability has been an ongoing concern for both new and long-established groups.

BREASTFEEDING GROUPS

Where the family is strong and not geographically scattered, it remains an important means of support for some breastfeeding women today. Yet today there may be a family history of one or more generations of artificial feeding or only short, token breastfeeding. The grandmothers and aunties may not have the experience of successful breastfeeding to share with the new mother. So an external support group may be a necessary adjunct to the family to help the mother continue to meet her baby's needs through breastfeeding (Figure 2.1). Indeed, the breastfeeding group has been described as a kind of surrogate grandmother (Thorley, 1983).

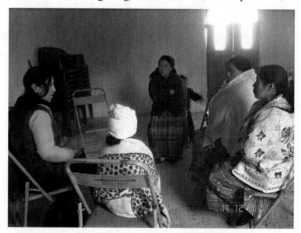

Figure 2.1. A mother-to-mother support group in Buena Vista, Totonicapán, Guatemala, facilitated by a peer counselor. Photo by Mimi Maza.

The first of these groups were the Nursing Mothers' Council, a California group founded in 1955, and La Leche League International (LLLI), founded by seven mothers in a suburb of Chicago in 1956 and soon to be worldwide (see Chapter 3) (Cowan, 2011; La Leche League, 1963, pp. 151-155; Prior, 1963). Unlike many in their community, the founding mothers had breastfed their babies and saw a need to provide support and information to other mothers. Other groups soon followed, such as the Nursing Mothers' Association (now the Australian Breastfeeding Association, ABA), founded by Mary Paton in Melbourne in 1964 (Thorley, 1990), and *Ammehjelpen*, founded by Elisabet Helsing in Norway in 1968 (see chapters 4 and 5). Derrick and Patrice Jelliffe summarized the emergence of mother support groups as being influenced by three factors of the time. The first was "a general reaction against the overemphasis on technology in modern life," the second, "a realization that health professionals … usually had little or no training (or much interest) in this field," and finally, an increasing awareness that artificial feeding could have negative consequences compared with the health-enhancing properties of human milk (Jelliffe & Jelliffe, 1978, p. 208). Today there are small and large groups in many countries, many of them affiliated with La Leche League International, others not.

Societal and technological changes in the last 34 years have moved the way self-help and mutual aid is sought and experienced beyond the often-quoted description provided by Alfred H. Katz and Eugene I. Bender (1976, p. 23), in which the face-to-face group was seen as the primary unit. Others have defined self-help organizations as operating independently of governments and receiving at least some of their support from sources other than government funding, and thus able to control their policies and how they operate (Donovan, 1977, p. 26). In a 1985 paper published posthumously, Alfred Katz summarized three key elements of self-help groups as fellowship, helping, and healing (Katz, 2003-2004). These elements no longer need face-to-face group settings to provide the support individuals seek. (The "healing" may be affective, such as an improvement in the mother's self-confidence.)

Whether electronic or face-to-face, the self-help and mutual aid experience usually involves the reaching out by the individual, even when contact is encouraged by another person. This applies whether the group is a Twelve Step one, such as Alcoholics Anonymous and GROW, or one of the myriad groups formed for mutual support. The group—online, face-to-face, or assisted by other technologies, such as social networking sites—is a potential means for the individual mother to receive the help she believes she needs. Through this the one, the individual, becomes part of the many, a member of a community linked by a common interest (Owen, 1978). Not only is support received and experience shared, but the mother also gains a perspective that she is not alone in her situation. The individual mother who desires to make personal changes (for instance, to learn how to follow her baby's feeding cues and not listen to negative friends) is enabled to work towards her goals through the support provided by group dynamics (Finn et al., 2009). For some mothers, the first encounter with the group takes courage, whether it is making the first telephone call or the physical act of walking in the door to the first meeting. This first experience will be affected by how welcoming the first contact is.

NEW MODES OF INTERACTION

Of course, face-to-face interaction, so eloquently described by Katz and Bender (1976), may not be how some participants experience the self-help group. This applies particularly to those physically isolated by transport difficulties, geographical factors, or the logistics of taking a baby out in inclement weather. For example, mothers of twins and triplets may feel particularly restricted. For mothers who are isolated, technology is increasingly providing access, with new developments bound to improve access even further in the future. Contact that is electronic, rather than face-to-face, may be the only way mothers of children with unusual breastfeeding challenges or rare disorders, and those with disabilities themselves, are able to find and interact with others who share a similar situation and concerns (Gribble, 2001; Madara, 1999-2000). Online groups are also attractive for busy people—and that includes mothers—because they provide "24/7 access to a concerned group of knowledgeable long-term friends" (Ferguson & the e-Patient Scholars Working Group, 2010, p. 59).

Charlotte Lombardo and Harvey Skinner have shown that online groups, as well as the traditional face-to-face group, meet the three "Functions of Self-Help Groups" that they have identified. These are: "Information sharing and experiential learning, social support, and empowerment and advocacy" (Lombardo & Skinner, 2003-2004).

Unless the individual has been provided with the URLs (website addresses) of relevant online groups, finding a suitable one may mean searching the vast firmament of Internet chatter for a relevant site, like astronomers searching for a distant star. For those who are not computer literate, this may be as daunting as walking in the door to the first meeting of a face-to-face group. Morton A. Lieberman (2003-2004) has described the importance of allowing members of online support groups to "lurk." That is, participate by reading messages without necessarily responding, as these members still feel a connection to the groups. Lurking also allows individuals to choose the group they are most comfortable with.

Use of Multiple Modes

Members of some self-help groups are able to experience interaction with the chosen group in a variety of modalities. Telephone or email counseling may be the first point of contact, even for those able to attend group meetings, and printed information and newsletters continue to fill a role in many mother support groups. Even if there are local discussion meetings, concerns may be discussed by telephone or email with an experienced member, or an online discussion board or chat room may provide some of the elements of a group discussion while the member sits at home. La Leche League International (LLLI) and the Australian Breastfeeding Association (ABA) are examples. Some organizations that provide face-to-face meetings and telephone support also post articles and the text of their leaflets on their websites, where individuals may download the information for themselves or for less computer-literate friends (Thorley, 2006). So for the individual, the experience of a self-help and mutual aid group may involve one or more of these elements and new modes provided by technologies yet to be developed.

Social networking sites such as Facebook muddy the waters somewhat as regards defining what a self-help group is, in that they facilitate interaction between individuals, even large groups of individuals; however, the primary purpose of such social networking sites is not self-help and mutual support. Nevertheless, some of the breastfeeding support groups include Facebook links on their websites. Young people, the demographic that includes young mothers, used social networking sites as their primary source of disaster and evacuation information during the 2010-2011 summer of disasters in Queensland, Australia. Thus mother support groups and health authorities would be wise to use these new media to provide short "bites" of information during disasters and evacuations to reassure breastfeeding mothers and to provide helpful tips and contact details. Unfortunately, even these media may be affected if the transmission towers are damaged or the electric power goes off and hand-held electronic devices cannot be recharged. Some examples of the use of multiple modes by support groups for the breastfeeding mother follow.

LLLI provides local meetings in many countries around the world, details of which can be searched on the main website (see chapter 3). Meetings in the local languages are often available, and written information on breastfeeding can be obtained from the League in a number of languages. Mothers can use the telephone or email to get local breastfeeding support from trained breastfeeding counselors in their local areas. They can also interact with other mothers by participating in the online forums in English or Spanish, with a trained breastfeeding counselor available.

The Australian Breastfeeding Association (ABA), formerly the Nursing Mothers' Association of Australia, provides face-to-face group meetings throughout Australia, as well as telephone counseling, email counseling, and a website. Antenatal breastfeeding classes for couples are also available. The website is regularly updated and provides downloadable information, the national breastfeeding helpline number accessible for the cost of a local call, a find-a-group facility, a contact process for email counseling, and a forum.

In Britain, the Association for Breastfeeding Mothers (ABM)[2] supports the formation of local mother support groups and its trained lay counselors provide counseling by telephone, email, or letter, with the emphasis on the immediacy of telephone counseling (ABM, 2010). It is one of several organizations providing support for breastfeeding women. The ABM website provides information about local breastfeeding support groups of all types, including La Leche League, Baby Cafés (see chapter 9), and drop-in centers.

Formation of Local Groups

Some of today's mother support groups are part of larger organizations, such as La Leche League International and the Australian Breastfeeding Association, and require prospective counselors to have successfully completed the required training and to adhere to the organization's standards and systems. Groups need to have a breastfeeding counselor in order to be established. Though smaller, the Baby Café concept is tightly controlled, so that only drop-in centers that measure up to the standards and are financially sustainable can use the title. Other mother support groups are purely local or form part of looser networks. The Association for Breastfeeding Mothers (ABM) provides the following information about forming local groups:

> The ABM encourages the formation of breastfeeding support groups to suit individual and local circumstances. It isn't necessary to be a counselor to start a support group, but trained

---

2   The initials "ABM" are also used for the Academy for Breastfeeding Medicine and artificial baby milks. In this chapter they refer to the Association for Breastfeeding Mothers.

counselors will often be happy to attend a group to offer support and information. Support groups can be a valuable source of contact for breastfeeding mothers. They offer mums an opportunity to meet and share experiences with other breastfeeding mums, expand their own knowledge of breastfeeding and widen their social circle. This can help when a new mum might be feeling isolated and out of touch with the world at large. We can offer advice to anyone wishing to set up a support group of their own.… (ABM, 2010).

Initially, mother support group founders and volunteer counselors have done their own administration, and some of the smaller or local groups still do this. As they grew, some of the larger associations with many groups needed administrative support to free counselors to meet the increasing demand for group activities and telephone counseling. Others manage with local volunteers. In a way, the ABM website serves as a kind of clearinghouse, putting mothers in touch with local breastfeeding support groups, which may otherwise have difficulty in becoming known, and providing advice on beginning a group.

Group Dynamics and Individual Experience

Within the modes of interaction available to members and intending members of self-help groups, the individual's experience of the group will be affected by how successful the organization is. However a group defines its success, if it is dynamic, welcoming of new members, and retains at least a core of ongoing members, it is likely to be attractive to the new member. These groups will have members flowing through them, new members joining, and some of the old members moving out of the group, but the group remains the repository of the collective experience, becoming more than a sum of its parts (Owen, 1978). Contrast this with the failing group or any group where new members are not welcomed by the long-term members who have formed a coterie, or where leaders are reluctant to close a group whose numbers have declined. A group whose meetings are too large for the intimacy of small-group interaction to be achieved may be daunting for some members, but meet the needs of those who attend for information, rather than participation.

Conclusion

As persons with a keen interest in self-help groups and/or self-care, it is easy for us to forget the age-old form of mutual support, which pre-dates the formal self-help movement and is still playing an important role. That is the family network, where it exists. Of course, for many who no longer have extended families or who live far from kin, the modern self-help group has taken on the role of a surrogate family. Support groups also assist those who cannot receive the help they need from others in the family, such as breastfeeding after a generation or more when breastfeeding was out of fashion. Working in our own areas of self-help, mother support, we are preoccupied by our own concerns. It is good to pause occasionally to "smell the roses," that is, to celebrate the diversity of this galaxy of helping modes of which mother support groups are a part.

Chapter Three

Mother Knows Best:
La Leche League

Kaye Lowman Boorom

No one noticed at the time, but something bold and daring took place in a small American town in the 1950s. Not even people living in the immediate area thought anything of it when a handful of women gathered in a living room in 1956 to talk. No one, not even the women in the room, realized that meeting would one day have worldwide ramifications and spawn a life-changing revolution that continues to impact people around the world nearly 60 years later.

They weren't plotting to overthrow a government or planning the unveiling of a scientific breakthrough. Quite the opposite. They were working within the establishment to undo much of what the modern science of the 1940s and 1950s had done. They were reclaiming birth and breastfeeding as nature had intended them to be, not as modern medical practices had reinvented them.

The women who began it all in 1956—Marian Tompson, Mary White, Edwina Froehlich, Betty Wagner, Mary Ann Cahill, Mary Ann Kerwin, and Viola Lennon—were, at the time, simply seven ordinary suburban mothers who gathered interested friends and neighbors to share their hard-earned knowledge about breastfeeding with other women who wanted to nurse their own babies, but lacked the information and support that were the critical components to enable them to succeed.

What happened next would be the stuff of legend if it hadn't actually happened. Seven housewives with the simple goal of sharing information with a handful of other women rose to the challenge of filling the enormous void they discovered. They went on to form a "club"—La Leche League, named after a shrine to the Spanish Madonna in St. Augustine, Florida: *Nuestra Senora de La Leche y Buen Parto* (Our Lady of Plentiful Milk and Happy Delivery). The name "La Leche" served as a code word of sorts since the word "breast" could not be said in polite company at the time. That modest local group quickly became an international organization that within little more than two decades was recognized as the world's leading resource for breastfeeding information.

How did it all happen? These seven radical thinkers took a decidedly un-radical approach to bringing about a revolution in birth and breastfeeding practices. Believing in their own instincts rather than the medical dictates of the day was more bold and daring than most of us who weren't raising children in the 1950s can comprehend. Doctors were all-knowing, never-to-be-questioned authority figures who told their patients what to do. And their patients, almost without exception, did exactly as they were told. That is, except for seven women living in a small Chicagoland suburb, and a few other brave souls like them scattered around the country. They dared to birth and nourish their babies "their" way, often enduring a lecture from the physician about the dire consequences of their decisions, or simply never told the doctor that they weren't following his orders.

Physicians of that era weren't alone in undermining a breastfeeding mother's confidence. Neighbors, mothers-in-law, and even complete strangers were quick to wonder aloud why anyone would want to be tied down to a nursing baby when the freedom provided by modern formula was so readily available. And, of course, the moment the baby cried, all of the naysayers were quick to assert that it was because the baby "wasn't getting enough" from his mother, who was already swimming against the social and medical current.

But unlike the Occupy Wall Street protesters of 2011 who took to the streets in their quest to bring about change, La Leche League's Founders succeeded in winning over converts to their cause by quietly telling their story to all who would listen, and letting their happy, healthy babies be the living proof that their way worked.

Word spread quickly about the new organization and those seven women who had information and answers to breastfeeding questions that no one else seemed to have. Soon 30 to 40 women, most of them people who had heard about the organization through friends of friends, were crowding into the monthly meetings at Mary White's house. When the living room was filled to capacity, women listened eagerly from the adjacent dining room, and none of the late-comers ever seemed to complain about having to park blocks away. The initial group quickly split into two groups to accommodate the unexpected, but nonetheless welcome crowds.

Friends told friends about La Leche League, and their friends told their friends, and on it went. With no money, no publicity, and no intention of reaching any further than their own neighborhoods, word of mouth brought a never-ending stream of new faces to the meetings and armloads of mail to Franklin Park from women who were too far away to attend meetings, but desperately wanted the information they needed in order to breastfeed their babies. First it was women in neighboring states who were writing and calling for help. But soon the ripples became tidal waves, and the calls and letters poured in from nearly every state in the country. The Founders were amazed at the hundreds of women who were looking to them for the information that could not be found anywhere else. The women at that first historic meeting at Mary White's house in 1956 could never have imagined the first group would explode into groups in over 70 countries, with more than 7,000 accredited Leaders by 2009.

Slowly at first, local newspapers began to take notice of the women and their mission. Headlines from the late 1950s and 1960s tell the story: "La Leche League Sponsors Meetings to Aid Mothers and Their Infants"; "League Tells Its April Schedule"; "Mothers Group for Breastfed Babies"; "Nursing Mothers Carry on Crusade"; "League Formed to Oppose Bottle Feeding of Babies, Reports Growing Support"; and even "The Womanly Art of Breastfeeding." Soon magazines began to take note of the women and their work. Articles appeared in *Baby Talk, Prevention,* and *Herald of Health* magazines, several Catholic publications, and a few medical journals. Word of mouth and ever-increasing magazine and newspaper publicity was generating 300 phone calls and 400 letters a month by early 1960.

The first national publicity came in the spring of 1960 from a feature in *Family Circle* magazine. That article alone generated 800 letters requesting breastfeeding help. The granddaddy of them all in terms of mail generated was an article in the May 1963 issue of *Reader's Digest*. Karen Pryor, a marine biologist from Hawaii, had written a book about breastfeeding based on her own experience and research she had done—including contacting the Founders of La Leche League (Pryor, 1963). Based on the friendship that blossomed with the Founders, she included a chapter about La Leche League, titled "They Teach the Joys of Breastfeeding." When that chapter was published in *Reader's Digest*, it gave La Leche League a level of exposure and credibility it had never had before. And the mail arriving daily in Franklin Park continued to grow exponentially.

Meanwhile, women who lived outside of Franklin Park began setting up La Leche League chapters in their own areas, at first in the United States, but soon spreading to the first "international" location in Canada. Volunteer mothers trained other mothers to become accredited Leaders of these groups. Before long, this mother support organization had spread worldwide. By the time the organization officially became La Leche League International in 1964, there were 115 groups in the United States and six in foreign countries.

No one, let alone young mothers with large families, could keep up with the explosive number of requests for breastfeeding information that arrived daily in the form of both letters and phone calls. Mary White answered many of the medically-related calls and letters, and her husband, Dr. Gregory White, graciously took the hundreds of long distance calls—a very expensive form of communication in those days—from distraught mothers with more complicated issues who could not find the help they needed anyplace else except from Dr. White. He never charged for his advice, and always made himself available, often at the expense of his own sleep.

But even with the addition of a small army of experienced nursing mothers who volunteered to answer the continuing onslaught of letters asking for breastfeeding information, it was impossible to keep up. So the Founders did what resourceful women have always done. They found a solution to the problem, in this case in the form of a "course by mail," in which they incorporated all of the information that they shared at the monthly meetings. They also created a monthly newsletter, with subscriptions available for $1.00 a year. Although Marian Tompson was the newsletter's editor for many years, it was Mary White, with her trusty red pen, who gave four decades of her life to reviewing nearly every word that La Leche League printed, always seeing to it that grammar and spelling were perfect and, most importantly, that every one of the hundreds and hundreds of La Leche League's newsletters, books, information sheets, and newspaper and magazine articles accurately reflected La Leche League's mission and philosophy. And, once again, Dr. White stepped up to volunteer his time to review all the La Leche League publications for medical accuracy.

The monthly newsletter stemmed the tide for a time, but the more mothers the Founders helped, the more they learned, and the more information they had to share. So in 1958 they wrote and printed the first version of *The Womanly Art of Breastfeeding*, a loose-leaf booklet. But even that turned out to be a stopgap measure, as the Founders' knowledge base continued to grow. Their next step was bold and daring: they decided to write a "real" book and pay to have it printed.

There were no deep pockets to reach into to fund the book, and bank-issued credit cards were still a thing of the future, so paying for the book was a daunting issue. But one thing the Founders were never short on was faith. So they arranged with the printer to pay for the books in installments, and then focused their attention on writing it.

As is often the case with bold and daring decisions, the Founders later admitted that they had no idea what they were getting into. They only knew that it was what they needed to do, and they plunged ahead. They met regularly to discuss ideas and share opinions about what should be included in the book. Each Founder worked on a section, and then they read and revised each others' work, rewrote, and revised again. The manuscript was reviewed for medical accuracy by two physicians who had extensive experience with breastfeeding mothers and babies.

The book was finally published four years and ten babies from the day it was started. The Founders needn't have worried about paying for the book's printing. The first press run—that happened the same month as the article in *Reader's Digest*—of 10,000 166—page books, priced at $3.00, sold out in less than two months, providing enough profit to pay the bill in its entirety and fund an immediate second printing. The rest, as they say, is history. The *Womanly Art of Breastfeeding* is now in its 8th revision.

Though much of La Leche League's growth and influence can be attributed to having the right people in the right place at the right time, equal credit must be given to the unique talents and abilities that each one of the Founders brought to the organization, as well as their wisdom in laying the necessary groundwork as each new challenge and opportunity came their way.

The bedrock they wisely built on was their partnership with two physicians who reviewed the *Womanly Art* for accuracy. These were Dr. Gregory White, husband of Founder Mary White, and Dr. Herbert Ratner, whose belief in the inherent wisdom of nature and his warm and wise parenting philosophy dovetailed so perfectly with the Founders' intuition about the importance of breastfeeding and a warm and responsive style of parenting. They were the trusted physicians who lovingly volunteered their time to review *The Womanly Art of Breastfeeding* for medical accuracy. These two remarkable men gave La Leche League and its Founders both credibility and an avenue for access to the medical establishment.

The medical establishment—ah, there was the rub. The 1940s and 1950s were a time of explosive medical advances, which along the way also enveloped birth and breastfeeding. Well-meaning doctors of the time were trained in the newest medical advances, including those that had moved childbirth out of the home and into the hospital. In the process, birth and breastfeeding became medical issues rather than natural events. Babies were wrested from anesthetized mothers under surgical lights in sterile operating rooms. Newborns were whisked off to a central nursery where they were cared for by a parade of strange nurses in starched uniforms rather than their own mothers. It logically followed that these babies should be fed the new "scientific" artificial formula rather than that old fashioned, unverifiable substance, their own mother's milk.

Many women knew in their hearts that this was not what they wanted for themselves or their babies. Yet it was the raw nerve and gritty determination of La Leche League's Founders and the women who joined them along the way that was responsible for bringing about the changes that have given women of today more control over their birth experience and the knowledge needed to breastfeed their babies.

Although there had always been a handful of supporters in the medical community—chief among them Dr. White and Dr. Ratner who understood and embraced the natural order of things—the majority of physicians in the 1950s, 1960s, and even into the 1970s believed that artificial formula out of a bottle was preferable to the unquantified substance that came from a mother's breasts.

It was a slow and often frustrating process to win over the medical establishment, or at least some sections of it. In La Leche League's early days, there were so few nursing mothers in the United States that there was little interest in studying human milk, and even less opportunity to find lactating women to study. Even so, every so often a research study would appear making some assertion about the quality (of lack thereof) of human milk, its nutrients (or lack thereof), or the reasons why "modern" women were unable to supply enough milk for their babies. Initially, Mary White began tracking these studies as they appeared in her husband's medical journals. It was Founder Marian Tompson who made it her life's work to delve into the studies, learning the protocols and educating herself, largely through one-on-one tutoring by Dr. Herbert Ratner, so that she could raise questions and determine the validity of the studies' results. A good deal of erroneous information, based on flawed study design, was making its way into medical journals and occasionally into the broader media. With the backing of Drs. White and Ratner, La Leche League began to contact both the researchers and the media to gently correct inaccurate information.

That, coupled with the ever-increasing number of women who were nursing their babies thanks to the information available through La Leche League, slowly began to turn the tide. By 2011 the percent of mothers in the United States who were breastfeeding their babies had jumped to nearly 75%, from the low of 20% recorded in 1956. In the most amazing turnaround of all, the American Academy of Pediatrics, who had been La Leche League's nemesis for so many years, endorsed breastfeeding as the preferred method of infant feeding in 1997. With no funding, no marketing savvy, and no goal other than to help their friends and neighbors, the seven women who banded together in 1956 and the influence of the organization they founded created a medical and cultural revolution.

How did they do it? They simply told their stories and shared their experiences with all who would listen. As Drs. White and Ratner began quietly opening doors within the medical community, the Founders gained an ever-widening audience for the knowledge they were eager to share— first at small, local medical meetings, then at state medical association meetings, hospitals, and medical schools. As La Leche League's reputation and credibility grew in the 1970s and '80s, Founder and longtime La Leche League President, Marian Tompson, found herself the invited guest speaker at congressional hearings, international health and nutrition organizations, and birth and breastfeeding symposiums in 33 countries around the globe. Today, at 82 years of age, Marian continues to be a relevant, sought-after speaker at home and abroad.

What began in Franklin Park, Illinois, in 1956 stands alone as perhaps the single most inspiring example of harnessing the power of women to challenge the status quo and upend medical practices from Alaska to Zimbabwe. Nearly every childbirth, breastfeeding, parenting, and infant nutrition organization that we know today has its roots in La Leche League and the La Leche League style of mother-to-mother support (Figures 3.1, 3.2, 3.3).

Figure 3.1. History of La Leche League

To read more about the history of La Leche League, see the following:

Cahill, M.A. (2001). Seven voices, one dream. Schaumburg, IL: La Leche League International.

Cowan, C. (2011). La Leche League. In A. O'Reilly (Ed.), The 21st century motherhood movement: Mothers speak out on why we need to change the world and how to do it. Toronto: Demeter Press.

Lowman, K. (2007). The revolutionaries wore pearls. Schaumburg, IL: La Leche League International.

Tompson, M.L., & Vickers, M.C. (2011). Passionate journey—My unexpected life. Amarillo, TX: Hale Publishing.

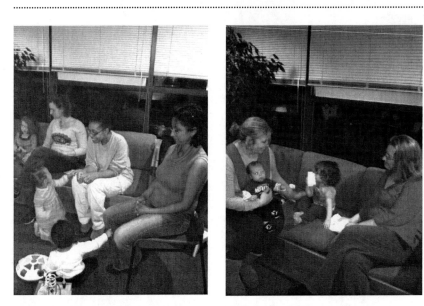
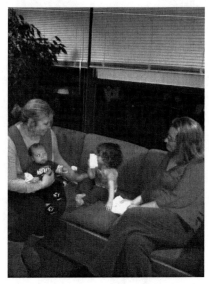

Figure 3.2. Mothers interacting with their children at a LLL meeting in the United States. Photo by Pam Freedman.

Figure 3.3. Mothers sharing their experiences at a LLL meeting in the United States today. Photo by Pam Freedman.

Part II: Mother Support Around the World: Examples

Chapter Four

Grassroots Mother Support as the Basis for a Large National Organization: The Australian Breastfeeding Association

Nina Berry, PhD

BACKGROUND

National and international bodies concerned with the health and nutrition of infants recommend exclusive breastfeeding for the first six months of a baby's life with remarkable unanimity (NHMRC, 2003; UK Department of Health, 2003; USDHHS, 2000; WHO/ UNICEF, 2003). Implicit in these recommendations is the recognition that the introduction of foods or fluids other than human milk before six months carries significant health risks.

Although the *Global Strategy for Infant and Young Child Feeding* recommends infants from six months of age "should receive nutritionally adequate and safe complementary foods while breastfeeding continues for up to two years of age or beyond" (WHO/ UNICEF, 2003, p. 8), many public health bodies in the developed world equivocate regarding total duration of breastfeeding (AAFP, 2001; AAP, 2005; NHMRC, 2003; Royal Australian College of Physicians, 2006; UK Department of Health, 2003). However, most public health bodies, including the Australian National Health and Medical Research Council, recommend infants continue to breastfeed after the introduction of table foods until at least the completion of the first year of life (NHMRC, 2003).

Nevertheless, relatively few infants anywhere in the world are fed according to the recommendations (Australian Bureau of Statistics, 2003; Bolling, Grant, Hamlyn, & Thornton, 2007; Centers for Disease Control, 2005; Statistics Canada, 2008). Even where most mothers begin breastfeeding, they also tend to terminate exclusive breastfeeding early and cease breastfeeding altogether well before the end of the first year of life. For example, only 60% of Australian mothers who begin breastfeeding continue even to six months, despite near universal initiation. Few mothers continue breastfeeding for 12 months or more and the proportion that continues to two years is negligible (Australian Bureau of Statistics, 2003). The pattern in similar in Canada where most mothers begin breastfeeding, but only 55% of them continue to six months, and very few mothers continue breastfeeding to 12 months (Statistics Canada, 2005). Although fewer American mothers initiate breastfeeding, most (84%) of those who do, continue to six months, but only a small proportion continue to 12 months (Centers for Disease Control, 2005). By six months only one in four British babies is breastfed (Bolling et al., 2007).

Many efforts to promote breastfeeding fail to acknowledge that in order to achieve the recommended infant feeding pattern, mothers must not only choose to initiate breastfeeding, but must choose to continue breastfeeding on a daily—and sometimes hourly—basis for many, many months. Furthermore, the decision to breastfeed or to continue breastfeeding is not made in isolation. Both the decision and the act occur within a social and cultural context.

Research

Research demonstrates that social support is associated with improved breastfeeding outcomes. Sikorski and colleagues' (2003) systematic review and meta-analysis identified a small but significant effect of support provided by healthcare professionals on overall breastfeeding duration, but no effect on duration of exclusive breastfeeding. However, mothers who receive the support of a trained community supporter were 1.5 times more likely to be breastfeeding exclusively at the final study assessment.

More recent trials confirm this finding. One study (Chapman, Damio, Young & Perez-Escamilla, 2004) conducted among low income American Latinas found that access to peer counseling services increased breastfeeding initiation and duration to three months. Another conducted in a socio-economically deprived area in the UK (Ingram, Rosser, & Jackson, 2005), found that the introduction of an initiative that included training peer supporters and establishing mother support groups improved breastfeeding prevalence in the area at eight weeks. Dennis and colleagues (2002) found that Canadian mothers who received telephone support from a trained peer were more likely to be breastfeeding and to be breastfeeding exclusively at three months postpartum.

Variation in the magnitude of the effect of mother support on breastfeeding outcomes are most likely explained by differences in the nature of the support intervention, the social milieu in which they are conducted (including birth and early feeding practices), and entrenched infant feeding patterns. There has been little, if any, analysis of the effect established mother support organizations might exert on breastfeeding prevalence over time, but one study suggests increases in breastfeeding prevalence followed increases in membership of the Australian Breastfeeding Association (then the Nursing Mothers' Association of Australia) (Smibert, 1989). It might be hypothesized that the establishment of groups such as LLLI, the Association of Breastfeeding Mothers, or the Australian Breastfeeding Association might have a multiplier as more mothers experience the support they offer and in turn offer support to those in their own peer groups.

Qualitative research is able to provide insight into the value of social support to breastfeeding mothers. McInnes and Chambers (2008) recently conducted a synthesis of qualitative research investigating mothers experiences and perceptions of breastfeeding support. Most mothers suggested that support from family or social networks was more important to them than support from healthcare providers.

However, a mother's social network or context may also be for her a source of confusion, self-doubt, and pressure to discontinue breastfeeding, particularly when friends or family members have limited breastfeeding knowledge or experience. McInnes and colleagues' (2008) work observed that even an extensive existing social support network did not guarantee support for breastfeeding. This finding is repeated in a number of other qualitative studies (including one from Australia), which also observe that mothers who wish to continue breastfeeding in the face of an unsupportive social network, frequently turn to mother support organizations to facilitate the creation of new, supportive social connections (Barona-Vilar, Excriba-Aguir, & Ferrero-Gandia, 2009; Gribble, 2008; Scott & Mostyn, 2003).

The qualitative findings are supported by quantitative research. A large study of American women found that those whose families supported artificial feeding were twice as likely to never initiate breastfeeding than those whose families supported breastfeeding (Khoury, Moazzem, Jarjoura, Carothers, & Hinton, 2005). This finding may be reflected in another study which found that a woman's level of comfort with the idea of formula feeding was a better predictor of breastfeeding intention than her level of comfort with the idea of breastfeeding (Nommsen-Rivers, Chantry, Cohen, & Dewey, 2010).

These results are congruent with the central tenets of Bandura's Social Learning Theory. Bandura (1977, p. 22) observed, "Most human behavior is learned observationally through modeling: from observing others, one forms an idea of how new behaviors are performed, and on later occasions this coded information serves as a guide for action." For first-time mothers, infant and young child feeding is a new behavior and, as such, vulnerable to the social milieu in which it occurs. Mothers have identified their experiences of others' infant feeding practices as important influences upon their own infant feeding decisions (Barona-Vilar et al., 2009; Ekstrom, Widstrom, & Nissen, 2003; Henderson, Kitzinger, & Green, 2000; Hoddinott & Pill, 1999).

The Role of Mother Support Organizations

Most women breastfeeding in the developed world do so within a cultural context that is not supportive of exclusive breastfeeding to six months and becomes less supportive of breastfeeding *per se* as the child grows (Gribble, 2008; McInnes & Chambers, 2008). In the absence of informal social support, mother support groups create a subculture that fosters breastfeeding and provides women with strategies for answering criticism and managing the often subtle, cultural pressures to stop breastfeeding or start inappropriate complementary feeding (Gribble, 2008; McInnes & Chambers, 2008). The support offered by mother support organizations may be particularly important where advice from healthcare providers is poor or does not support the mother's desire to continue breastfeeding (McInnes & Chambers, 2008).

Mother support organizations offer a variety of services to new mothers. However, they are all founded on the provision of informational support by trained, and usually experienced, lay breastfeeding counselors, either by telephone, email, or face-to-face. Perhaps more importantly, most of these groups facilitate the formation of breastfeeding supportive social networks, either through group meetings or Internet-based social networking tools, such as Facebook or purpose-built Internet fora.

The Australian Context

Australia is a constitutional democracy, a member of the British Commonwealth. It has three tiers of government: Federal, State, and local. Australia's population is currently estimated to be approaching 22.5 million people, and there are close to 300,000 births in Australia annually. Citizens and permanent residents have universal access to healthcare, which is delivered by the State Government Departments of Health and funded through Federal income and consumption taxes. Primary healthcare and screening are generally provided to mothers and babies by public health nurses (Child and Family Health Nurses or Maternal and Child Health Nurses) free of charge in local clinics. These clinics are generally administered by State departments of health, although in Victoria, they are the purview of local government. From these clinics mothers and babies can be referred to general practitioners (family physicians) and specialists, including pediatricians and allied healthcare providers. These services can be provided at no cost to the consumer.

Working Australian mothers have long been entitled to 12 months unpaid maternity leave. More recently, a Paid Parental Leave Scheme has been introduced, in addition to the unpaid leave. This Scheme entitles a newborn or newly adopted child's primary caregiver to 18 weeks of leave paid at the National Minimum Wage ($589.40 gross per week at the time of writing).

THE AUSTRALIAN BREASTFEEDING ASSOCIATION

The Australian Breastfeeding Association was established in 1964 as the Nursing Mothers' Association (and later the Nursing Mothers' Association of Australia). Initially the invention of six women, led by Mary Paton, the Association has grown from a small grassroots mother-to-mother support organization to one that attracts significant Federal funding for specific programs. Paton established the Association in response to her own struggle to find the support she needed to breastfeed her own children (Reiger, 2001).

Probably as a result of this personal experience, Paton's insight into the needs of mothers who wished to breastfeed their children was remarkable, even prescient. She envisaged an Association that would stand in the place of supportive extended families and/or social networks. From its inception, the Association focused on providing mother-to-mother support through informal local group meetings and, later, telephone counseling. It differed from La Leche League International in that it explicitly maintained breastfeeding as its primary, if not sole, focus, avoiding the League's more prescriptive application of a philosophy of total motherhood—a philosophy which led the League to struggle with supporting mothers who were employed outside the home during the 1980s (Blum & Vanderwater, 1993). Paradoxically, maintaining such a strict focus on breastfeeding allowed local groups the flexibility to respond to the needs and lifestyles of the mothers they served (Reiger, 2001).

The founding mothers, as they are known, sought to create an independent organization with a tight National structure that has been described as emanating from the local group like the spokes of a wheel. A group cannot be established unless and until a trained volunteer breastfeeding counselor (or, more recently, a community educator) is available to facilitate it (Reiger, 2001). These volunteers all receive training, not only in breastfeeding support, but they must become familiar with—and undertake to comply with—the Association's founding document, the Code of Ethics. This requirement has ensured that, although each group has a local flavor, the Association has retained a coherent identity.

It was—and is—evolutionary rather than revolutionary in its approach, requiring volunteers to foster and protect relationships, not only between themselves and the mothers they serve, but also between the Association and healthcare providers. This provision, given expression in the Code of Ethics, reflects a desire on the part of the founding mothers that the Association be a source of education and information for healthcare professionals as well as the community (Reiger, 2001).

Today's Association currently offers a 24-hour National Breastfeeding Helpline staffed entirely by volunteers who hold Nationally Recognized Qualifications in Breastfeeding Education (Counseling), email counseling, an Internet forum and website that contains a large amount of breastfeeding information, a retail arm, local group meetings where mothers may access face-to-face counseling and support, access to local breastfeeding counselors, ante-natal education, health professional education, including conferences and seminars, and several publications, including a glossy magazine that is mailed to members six times a year. The Association also produces and sells its own *meh tai* style baby sling, accredits baby care rooms in the community, administers the Baby Friendly Workplace Accreditation scheme, and encourages local businesses to demonstrate their support for breastfeeding by displaying a "Breastfeeding Welcome Here" sticker that also includes a large ABA logo.

Since 2005, the Australian Breastfeeding Association has been a Registered Training Organization, developing and delivering Nationally Recognized Qualifications in Breastfeeding Education (Counseling and Community) and in Training and Assessment. This has been made possible by significant federal funding, the result of many years of dedicated lobbying by the Association's volunteers and staff.

In addition to these community activities, the Association actively lobbies both Federal and State Governments and has been instrumental in the development of two National Breastfeeding Strategies (in 1995 and 2010) and several state breastfeeding policies, which mandate the protection, promotion, and support of breastfeeding within state health services. The Association was also instrumental in establishing the National Paid Parental Leave Scheme. The Australian Breastfeeding Association is one of the most successful mother support organizations in the world, with around 15,000 members–possibly the highest per capita membership prevalence seen in any country in the world–and around 1450 volunteer breastfeeding counselors and community educators.

However, the Australian Breastfeeding Association faces a number of challenges as we move farther into the 21st Century. In the face of an aging population and reduced taxation base, successive governments have taken steps to increase workforce participation, particularly among women. This has, in turn, resulted in a dwindling volunteer workforce, as mothers tend to return to paid employment sooner than they once did. Simultaneous increases in the expectations placed upon the Association's volunteers in response to the accountabilities created by service agreements that accompany government grants have the potential to overburden the volunteer workforce. Although Mary Paton eschewed professionalization because the accountabilities such a model brings inevitably result in the sacrifice of some degree of independence, this may be unavoidable if the Association is to avoid becoming a victim of its own success.

In addition, the current generation of mothers appears to prefer a more spontaneous, "drop-in" style delivery for face-to-face breastfeeding support. Furthermore, they tend to be more comfortable in the world of online social networking, requiring the Association to rethink established systems and structures. These mothers seem to be less interested in "joining" established social groups or networks, rather preferring the perception that they have created (or perhaps collected) their own networks. The rise of online social networking, compounded by the speed at which the nature of online social networking reworks and re-invents itself, will require the Association to develop new skill sets and consider new strategies to meet the rising costs associated with maintaining an online presence.

In spite of the Association's achievements and the founding mothers' almost prescient commitment to mother support as foundational in the fight to reverse the cultural shift towards artificial feeding, it should be noted that breastfeeding prevalence beyond the first weeks of life has remained stable in Australia for over a decade and a half and the use of infant formula by breastfeeding mothers has increased (Amir & Donath, 2008; Australian Bureau of Statistics, 2003; Donath & Amir, 2002). Support for breastfeeding, including that provided by mother support organizations, cannot alone create environments that support breastfeeding. Such supportive environments will be characterized by a suite of measures that include, but are not limited to, regulation of commercial and industrial conditions; universal access to timely, skilled breastfeeding support; and the protection of birth practices that facilitate the establishment of strong breastfeeding relationships.

Chapter Five

The Scandinavian Breastfeeding Adventure: The First Years (1968–78)

Elisabet Helsing, Dr.Med.Sci.

PERSONAL HISTORY

As a young Scandinavian mother in 1965, I have to confess that I was not particularly interested in breastfeeding. Of course, I myself breastfed, that was the done thing. And I was first mildly surprised, then irritated, at the doublespeak of the nurse at the health station, who gave me for free two little satchels of infant formula saying, "Of course, breast is best, but should you not have enough milk, these are nice to have." Not enough milk? Never struck me as the remotest possibility. But as time went by and I spoke with young co-mothers in my vicinity, I learned otherwise. Even the official literature distributed to mothers at the health station gave little encouragement: "Relatively few mothers," it was stated, "indeed only some 30 percent of the total, produce sufficient milk to carry their babies through the entire period of breastfeeding…" (Njå, 1965). That set off my "breastfeeding career."

Why was I different, having no problems with breastfeeding? For one thing, I apparently belonged to the lucky 30 percent who "had enough." But why? One of my friends provided a further clue, "I, too, 'lost' my milk during a bad bout of flu," said she. "But I refused to accept it, so I put him to the breast incessantly and hey, presto! The milk came back." It sounded like a miracle: could it be that the loss of milk was *reversible*? Very interesting. Being by nature a curious person, I started reading up on the subject.

THE U.S. SETS AN EXAMPLE

I soon stumbled across a slim blue book with the (in my opinion) somewhat romanticized title: *The Womanly Art of Breastfeeding*. This book, however, had it all: the why, what, and how of breastfeeding, told in simple words.

A few newspaper articles and radio performances on my part later, it was becoming clear to me that those who maintained that modern mothers were not interested in feeding their offspring in the old-fashioned way were dead wrong. The articles I wrote resulted in a flood of letters from mothers, letters full of tears, sad tales, and queries about breastfeeding. I found myself repeating the same points over and over again, and eventually I started writing them down.

Latching on (to stay with the vocabulary) to the ideas expressed in the little blue book, and noting that the organization behind the book, La Leche League International, might have room for a group in Norway, I wrote to them. I soon received an answer from Edwina Froehlich, one of the LLL Founders, welcoming me into the organization. First, however, there were some formalities, which, much to my chagrin at the time, were never completed, since the LLL mother charged with the admission of new members from abroad had had a baby and, therefore, never had the time to complete my application. Sound familiar?

Unstoppable Scandinavians

Not to be stopped, I decided to establish an organization myself, independent of others. Including me, I had ten mothers who had declared their willingness to help other mothers. We called ourselves *Ammehjelpen* (Amme = breastfeed, hjelpen = help) and with incredible speed, or so it seemed to the initiators, the organization grew and spread. None of us had experience in organizing, and all of us worked for free. It never struck any one of us that it could be otherwise. Ammehjelpen was established in October 1968, and became, to my later knowledge, the third mother-to-mother support group created globally. In 1973 Sweden followed suit when *Amningshjälpen* was formed. Just as they chose a name very similar to the Norwegian one, the organizational structure was quite similar in the Swedish and the Norwegian movement, but the recruitment of "help mothers" was a little different. In Sweden, the mothers recruited were more often what may be termed "alternative." There seemed to be, for example, a higher percentage of vegetarians in Amningshjälpen than in the population in general. Unfortunately, the Swedish organization never got the support from the health authorities that Ammehjelpen enjoyed in Norway. For example, when a ministerial "Expert Committee on Breastfeeding" was established in 1973 in Sweden and in 1974 in Norway, the Swedish committee had one person out of 13 representing mothers (and she was by chance Norwegian). The Norwegian committee had four mother representatives out of 14. The secretary of the committee was from

Ammehjelpen and wrote much of the text in the recommendations of the group.

In Denmark the organizational picture seemed to be more varied. An important difference was that the Danish mother-to-mother support group, corresponding to the Swedish and Norwegian ones, had been led by a La Leche League member since 1974. They called themselves "*Ammehjælpen, associated with LLLI.*" In 1981 they were one of several organizations in Denmark providing mother-to-mother support in breastfeeding. An organization primarily formed to improve birthing conditions, under the name *Parents & Birthing,* had a sub-group named *The Breastfeeding Counseling Group*, which was a mother-to-mother support group. Finally, small projects such as "*Mother Earth*" and "*Women's association for developing countries, the group on breastfeeding,*" were also established.

Projects Versus Movements

At this point it may be useful to make a distinction: since mother-to-mother support groups are new to most societies, they will be looked upon as interventions. Any discussion of "interventions," however, should distinguish between *projects* and *movements*.

Ideally, *projects* are of limited duration—they have a starting point and a termination date. Projects are planned in advance and may or may not be open to adjustment under way. Projects are usually very dependent on resources from outside the project area—material as well as human resources. Problems and solutions are usually defined by well-meaning outsiders, not by those with the problems targeted for support, the problem owners.

Ideally, *movements* are first and foremost characterized by control over priorities and actions by those who have the problem. The ideas behind a movement may well come from outside the movement itself, but the ideas take time to grow and mature and become adjusted to the local reality. The problem owners formulate their views about problems, priorities, and solutions. There is no fixed plan available a long time in advance, although good movements need both planning and analysis; movement leaders first have to use their intuition to feel their way forward. Intuition is an important tool for understanding the exceedingly complex situation which problems taken up by a movement usually play. This requires intimate knowledge of the problems, as well as their causes. Movement leaders need to understand not only what is said and expressed openly, but also what is behind the words and under the surface.

Movements take their own time and have no defined time frame. Their exact starting point may be difficult to grasp, and so may their end. Either they peter out and die, or they are suppressed (as is very often the case), or they grow and lead to social change. The latter may be the most significant aspect of movements versus projects: the great potential of movements for social change. This was what we saw and experienced as regards breastfeeding in those heady first years. In order to survive, the mother-to-mother support had to be expressed and organized as a movement, not a project.

MOTHER SUPPORT OR MOTHER-TO-MOTHER SUPPORT

In retrospect, I personally see a distinction between mother support (MS) and mother-to-mother support (MtMS) groups. The BFHI Step 10 is not much help in clarifying this distinction since it does not give a clear definition of what is meant by *"Foster the establishment of breastfeeding support groups and refer mothers to them on discharge from the hospital or clinic."* As we found out the hard way, health workers should not be expected to start MtMS groups. Too many attempts at doing that, however well meaning, have failed simply because the health workers were trying and failing to act on behalf of the problem-owners, the mothers.

It is very desirable that health workers and MtMS groups are on good terms and work together. It would be highly undesirable if these potential helpers of mothers should see one another as enemies.

It might be helpful to go back to the basic question: *"What is breastfeeding?"* A great many women with breastfeeding problems are helped solely by being asked: "What would you have done with your breastfeeding problem if you had been cast off with your baby on a deserted island?" Most, but not all, breastfeeding problems are simple. Helping a mother requires empathy, but not enormously much in the way of training. But as we know, humans are tricky things, and a few will need specialist support. Then the lactation specialists enter the scene, and we are no longer talking about mother-to-mother support, but rather about a specialized form of mother support. Mother support can have as many expressions as there are facets to breastfeeding. Just a few examples are:

- Maternity protection legislation supports mothers.
- Baby-Friendly Hospitals support mothers.
- Prohibition of infant formula marketing supports mothers.
- Mother-to-mother support supports mothers.
- IBCLC support supports mothers.

- Evidence-based material on breastfeeding in practice supports mothers.
- Etc., etc., etc.

BACK TO SCANDINAVIA

The Scandinavian countries are, in spite of appearances to the contrary, quite different. Table 5.1, for example, shows the differences in live births 1996-2000, that is, potentially breastfed babies in the three Scandinavian countries. Sweden is by far the largest of the three.

Table 5.1. Average number of live births annually in the Scandinavian countries 1996–2000

Country	Live Births
Denmark	66,951
Norway	58,522
Sweden	90,688

Source: NOMESCO (Nordic Medico-Statistical Committee). (2005). *Health statistics in Nordic countries 2003.* Copenhagen: NOMESCO.

As the years went by, the example of LLLI continued to be important to the Scandinavian groups, but in the Norwegian Ammehjelpen, we still felt it necessary to retain our independence. There were several reasons for this. The North American material, when translated to Norwegian, looked odd. There was nothing wrong with the factual information; it was the presentation that was distinctly un-Norwegian. But this did not deter us from using existing organizational ideas and practical knowledge whenever we came across it. At that time publications on practical aspects of breastfeeding, however, were few and far between, but we used the little there was. Apart from the LLL material, our mentors were the Jelliffes, Illingworth, Applebaum, and the Newtons,[3] among others. As time went by, the trickle of information on breastfeeding and human milk swelled to the present deluge, where one can indulge in the luxury of picking out the best. Evidence-based material in quite specialized areas is also available now.

Organizations and Organizing

Few of the Scandinavian initiators had any organizational experience. This was reflected in a rather experimental attitude to organizing. The advantage of this experimentation was that a model might be found that suited this

---

3   Note: Dr. Derrick B. Jelliffe, Mrs E.F. Patrice Jelliffe, Dr. Richard M. Applebaum, and Drs. Michael and Niles Newton were leading breastfeeding advocates who were important sources of information and support to the new mothers' groups. [Editors]

particular group of organizing citizens: mainly young mothers with babies and small children. The disadvantage was that experimentation invariably leaves some people disappointed, and much time is used in discussing and trying out models that fail.

One particular trait that seemed to repeat itself in many of the Mother-to-Mother Support groups was the basic structure. There had to be leadership, but quite a lot of effort went into seeing to it that the structure did not become hierarchical. This might be a more or less conscious effort to avoid a "male" organizing pattern in organizations that necessarily would be female-dominated. This being 1969-1970, there was a strong influence from the feminist movement, and many of us were doubling as feminists and *ammehjelpers* ("help mothers"). In Norway we had no problems in explaining this double loyalty: the problem as we saw it was not at all with breastfeeding or not breastfeeding. There is really no alternative to the breast, just as there is no alternative to the uterus. The question was not whether or not to breastfeed, but rather whether or not to have babies. If we went in for procreation, this meant taking the whole package, so to speak.

In the MtMS groups, many questions arose as the membership grew: What should be the criteria for allowing a woman to become a counselor in the framework we provided? Could men be members? Could women who had not breastfed be members? What were the limits to our advice—should we include other aspects of infant feeding or rearing? Birthing? Do we really need something as formal as a constitution? How do we keep in touch with new developments and research? How do we keep in touch with each other? How will the modern means of communication influence the way we interact with mothers? With one another? The answers to these many questions would vary from country to country, from group to group. They would vary with the initiators and the support the initiators were able to drum up.

Something to Read

As mentioned above, I found myself writing the same advice to mothers over and over again, since the problems mothers had were of similar origin (often brought on by misinformation and thoughtless remarks). LLLI had a "hospital brochure" for use right after birth. I translated it and adapted it to our realities. To cut a long story short, I then went to our Directorate of Health with the draft brochure and met a kindred spirit in Dr. Gro Harlem Brundtland who immediately saw its importance.

Initially, however, a number of health professionals resisted the idea that mere mothers should be allowed to express themselves on the subject of breastfeeding on behalf of the Directorate of Health. Sense however prevailed, and in early 1969, after having been vetted by all who were presumed to have anything to say on the matter, the brochure was ready. It turned out that there was a constant demand for the little printed matter, not least from the health workers. It was repeatedly reprinted, and today 2 million copies have been issued, which means that all primiparas may have been given a copy in the maternity ward. It has grown over the years, from 12 pages in 1969 to 40 pages today. The small booklet was written "*by mothers for mothers*": this was the *problem owners* speaking up, defining their problem.

A small book was the next project. I had some difficulty in finding a publisher, being constantly met with the incredulous "a whole book about breastfeeding? That is not possible!" But it turned out to be not only possible, but the book was a bestseller. Eventually, 70,000 copies were printed.

Health Workers and Ammehjelpen

How did health professionals receive professional breastfeeding mothers? Again we have to turn to the familiar terrain of Norway for evidence from real life.

By the mid-1970s, Ammehjelpen had about 500 active "help mothers," as they called themselves at that time. With 50,000 to 60,000 births per year and each counselor having from five to 10 contacts per year, about five to 10 percent of mothers with babies contacted Ammehjelpen at one point in time.

This hardly meant that Ammehjelpen threatened the established health system. Still, the fact that mothers started to organize in order to teach each other how to breastfeed initially puzzled and sometimes annoyed health workers. It seemed to indicate that they had failed in what they considered one of their areas of responsibility—and this was true, to some extent. Although breastfeeding was *encouraged* in the maternity wards, it was not actually *taught*. This being before the IBCLCs (lactation consultants) came on the scene; it was not readily acknowledged that breastfeeding was a subject worthy of teaching. Being the author of several books about the subject, I have often had to explain myself to incredulous listeners who exclaim, "Come on—don't tell me that you have written a whole book about *breastfeeding* …? Ha, ha, ha!"

In the beginning, therefore, Ammehjelpen often had to appear as critics—of the system, of misinformation from individual health workers, and of misleading statements from the baby food industry. The organization had not chosen this role for itself; its aim was teaching those who wanted to be taught. And the remuneration to the ammehjelpers has continued to be the apparently deeply felt gratitude of those who succeed in something that meant a lot to them, depicted in the dry statistics below (Table 5.2).

Table 5.2. Breastfeeding in Scandinavia During the First Year of Life

Full breastfeeding (%)			Partial breastfeeding (%)	
Country	1st week	4 mos.	6 mos.	6 mos.	12 mos.
Denmark 1995	86	60	17	61	18
Norway 1998/99	96	44	7	80	36
Sweden 1997	94	69	42	74	

Source: NOMESCO (Nordic Medico-Statistical Committee). (2005). *Health statistics in Nordic countries 2003*. Copenhagen: NOMESCO.

Chapter Six

Mother Support in Malaysia

Siti Norjinah Moin
Local Governance Coordinator for WABA

BACKGROUND

The *Persatuan Penasihat Penyusuan Ibu Malaysia* (PPPIM), or the Malaysian Breastfeeding Association, is a voluntary non-profit organization founded in October 1974. It started with a group of women who were concerned about the decline in breastfeeding and the lack of information to support mothers wishing to breastfeed. The prime objective of the Association is to encourage and assist mothers and to make available support information through telephone and discussion.

From a small gathering of breastfeeding mothers meeting every first Wednesday of each month, it has become an association with five chapters in five different states. These are Selangor, Kuala Lumpur, Ipoh, Penang, and Kuantan. It was registered as the *Persatuan Penasihat Penyusuan Ibu Selangor* (Selangor Breastfeeding Association). Each group was headed by foreigners married to expatriates working in Malaysia (who were members of LLLI and the NMAA) and a small number of local women. To garner funds they set up fundraising events by having jumble sales, garden fetes, and car boot sales.[4] Local mothers joined the group through word of mouth. During this time most mothers were mixed-feeding or totally formula feeding. Mothercraft nurses from milk companies were making their rounds, visiting and giving free samples to new mothers. In every clinic and hospital, samples were easily available. Indirectly, the medical professionals were agents and promoters of formula milk companies.

The urban women have often moved from their families to work in the city, thus removing them from their extended families. Mostly their elders or family members would be present during their early days postpartum, but

---

4   "Car boot" sales are similar to garage sales or yard sales in other countries, that is, sales of second-hand items.

all too soon the new mothers were not receiving very much encouragement from their own mothers and mothers-in-law. This is due to the fact that many of those born in the 1950s and 1960s were bottle-fed, and they were not exposed to proper breastfeeding. They considered breastfeeding inconvenient compared to bottle-feeding. Moreover, new mothers only have 42 days of maternity leave, and their babies may have problems when they go back to work.

Meanwhile, members were getting calls from new mothers wanting help with early breastfeeding. They started doing their rounds of home and hospital visits. Hospitals welcomed members to help out in the postnatal wards. Indeed it was helpful for a mother to be put in touch with another mother who had a similar experience. The breastfeeding decision and its potential success depend very much on the information, support, and encouragement a mother receives when she needs it most. Our meetings where mothers meet other mothers and are able to exchange experiences and information proved to be an encouraging factor. Seeing another mother successfully breastfeeding and learning to cope with early initiation of breastfeeding tend to make mothers more confident and able to breastfeed longer. They found that this particularly helped them to face criticism from relatives and friends who may not understand why they chose to breastfeed.

Our members and Breastfeeding Counselors were better able to deal with hospital routines that may have a negative effect on breastfeeding. For example, they encouraged having babies "room-in" with their mothers, with no "introduction to formula feeding." The assurance that they belonged to a mother-to-mother support group with established principles and beliefs made the new mothers feel less intimidated in a professional atmosphere. Overcoming this situation of negative hospital routines helped both the medical professionals and the breastfeeding volunteer to combine their efforts toward a common goal. This was before the Baby-Friendly Hospital Initiative.

Members were given training to become certified Breastfeeding Counselors following some of the NMAA and LLLI guidelines. We have our own training modules for our Breastfeeding Counselors. We have our own mobile libraries where members are able to get more information on breastfeeding and mothering. The association distributed leaflets covering various topics relating to early initiation and how to keep and store milk for working mothers. In 1979 we had our first seminar on breastfeeding with Dr. Hugh Jolly from England as our guest speaker. In the same year, we became a national association known as *Persatuan Penasihat Penyusuan Ibu Malaysia* (PPPIM), or the Malaysian Breastfeeding Association.

Barriers Encountered

In the early 1980s, we were losing our expatriate members, as more locals were taking over when the contracts of foreign members' husbands expired. Companies were not engaging foreigners because of the economic "slow down." Locals were not able to do full time volunteer work, as most women were, and still are, in the workforce. The media and advertisements of products for artificial feeding were a hindrance to our breastfeeding work. With no office as base except "home to home," we were facing a difficult time in promoting breastfeeding. Health professionals in hospitals also changed when the older ones retired or transferred to other states. New heads were working with milk manufacturers; thus we were heading for a "brick wall" with no financial support.

New Opportunities

We changed our strategy in 1984 by joining other volunteer organizations like the Malaysian Council for Child Welfare (MCCW). Being on the Executive Committee of the MCCW and helping out with their activities, like the International Children's Day celebration, has helped us to gain allies and link with the Ministry of Health, Ministry for Social Welfare, WHO, UNICEF, and other voluntary organizations. The president of the MCCW was the Minister for Social Welfare and Family Development, Datin Paduka Zaleha Ismail, and the Vice President was the chief of the Paediatric Institute, Dr. Mohd Sham Kasim. With these two important figures as our mentors, breastfeeding was heading to a bright light at the end of a tunnel. We participated in various health fairs, exhibitions, and gave counseling in hospitals and community events.

The International Baby Food Action Network (IBFAN) and International Organisation for Consumer Union (IOCU) in Penang, spearheaded by Annelies Allain and Anwar Fazal, invited us to the IBFAN Forum in 1989 in Manila. Meeting and getting to know other global breastfeeding movements was an eye opener, thus the encouragement that we are not alone supporting breastfeeding. We brought home the knowledge that there is training by Wellstart on breastfeeding management. Thus we encouraged the Ministry of Health to send a team of delegates to be trained by Dr. Audrey Naylor. With trained health professionals, it would make it easier for us to work with the Ministry of Health. They eventually sent a team comprised of a pediatrician, an obstetric gynecologist, and a nutritionist in 1993.

In 1991, Anwar Fazal introduced Sarah Amin and the newly formed World Alliance for Breastfeeding Action (WABA), based in Penang. We had our first World Breastfeeding Week in 1992 with the theme "Baby Friendly." Following this event, UNICEF and WHO launched the Baby-Friendly Hospital Initiative (BFHI).

In 1992, using the IBFAN training module, we developed the 32-hour breastfeeding management course. Local breastfeeding practices were added to suit our requirement. Thirty of our breastfeeding counselors and selected health professionals from the public hospitals attended this training. The following year we were invited by the Family Health Division of the Ministry of Health to assist them with the 18-Hour BFHI training for their core trainers.

In 1994 the Ministry of Health launched their BFHI during the World Breastfeeding Week celebrations in the Kuala Lumpur General Hospital. Our Queen, Tuanku Bainun, at the same time graciously officiated at the opening of our Breastfeeding Room in the Maternity Hospital.

In 1994, the association was put to task to organize the regional training for UNICEF/WHO's 40-hour "Counseling: A Training Course." This was funded by the Regional UNICEF office in Bangkok. Thirty medical professionals from Myanmar, Indonesia, and Malaysia were trained by Dr. Felicity Savage who was working for WHO at the time. Later, in 1996, we trained the trainers of the Institute of Public Health on the 40-hour counseling training. Following this our members were also trained as BFHI national assessors and were added to the Ministry of Health team.

Using the platform of the Baby-Friendly Hospital Initiative and World Breastfeeding Week, we now have many trained Breastfeeding Counselors in all 14 states in Malaysia. The movement was expanding with the support of the Ministry of Health and UNICEF, but there was not much financial support. We managed to pull resources to train these Breastfeeding Counselors. WABA has consistently supported us by providing materials and by putting us into the international breastfeeding scene.

Together with WABA we launched the Maternity Protection campaign in 2000, preparing for the International Labor Organization Convention in 2002. Working together with the Malaysian Trade Union Congress, the National Congress Women's Organisation, and the Malaysian Council for Child Welfare, we created awareness and asked for more maternity leave for women. It was a long process, asking for an increase from 28 weeks to 36 weeks of paid maternity leave. In 2010 this was accepted and adopted by parliament.

By 2003 we had 118 public hospitals designated as Baby-Friendly in Malaysia, making us third in the world next to Sweden and Oman. This is a great achievement to us, as we are part of the 10th Step of the BFHI through providing mother support. Every two years these hospitals are reassessed. The association sits on several committees of the Ministry of Health: the National Breastfeeding Committee, the Code of Ethics on Infant Formula Products, the Codex Alimentarius Committee, the Food Security and Labeling Committee, and the Disciplinary Committee on the Code of Ethics, to name a few.

There are now 133 Baby-Friendly Hospitals in the country; and three public and 177 private hospitals are yet to be accredited. We are targeting at least 35 private hospitals to take up the initiative, as more mothers are going there to deliver daily. By doing this, we can have higher breastfeeding rates. We are also working on sustaining the BFHI and getting more mothers to exclusively breastfeed until six months and continue until two years and beyond.

After 10 years of celebrating World Breastfeeding Week, we are reflecting on what we have done so far for breastfeeding here (Figures 6.1 and 6.2). Now we have on-line breastfeeding support groups, our very own Facebook page, Breastfeeding Mother-to-Mother Support, Breastfeeding Information Bureau: Get Your Facts Right, the Breastfeeding Advocates Network, Kumpulan Ibu2 Menyusu (Breastfeeding Mothers' Group), and the Natural Parenting: Father Support Group. Other breastfeeding agencies include the Breastfeeding Information Bureau or BIB Malaysia, BIB Consultancy, and Susuibu.Com.

Today, we stand tall on breastfeeding support in this country, after starting with a catalyst group of mothers in their effort to encourage women to breastfeed. The emphasis is on "mother-to-mother" support, training breastfeeding counselors, and training health professionals. We are the focal and referral point for breastfeeding matters in this country and the region.

In conclusion, sustaining a "mother-to-mother support group" without any grants or financial backing can be very difficult. Project funding is only available for a one-time basis, and most of the time it is not sufficient to cover the hidden costs. Breastfeeding counselors move on when their children grow and wean off the breast. We have to find new members and continue to train new counselors. This cycle has kept on repeating over the three decades of our existence as an organization. There is no compensation or allowances for volunteer service. Many a time, members shy away after a period, and the counseling service is being watered down. Only the strong, dedicated, and passionate remain to hold on.

If breastfeeding mother-to-mother support is to remain as the 10th step of Baby-Friendly Hospital Initiative, then WHO and UNICEF should look into this seriously. The country must be aware of the plight that volunteer groups like us are going through with much difficulty to help sustain the BFHI in their country. We cannot say "no" or turn away mothers in need of help at a critical time. Putting us at the 10th Step is like pushing the bulk without even batting an eye; it is like pushing a great weight while seeming calm.

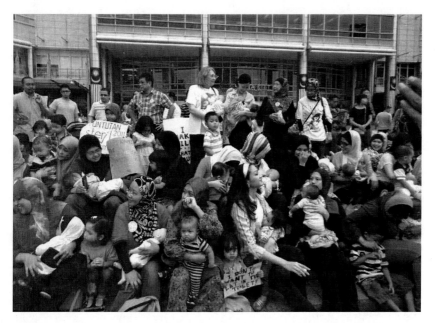

Figure 6.1. Section of the crowd at the FlashMob event in Kuala Lumpur for World Breastfeeding Week, August 2011.

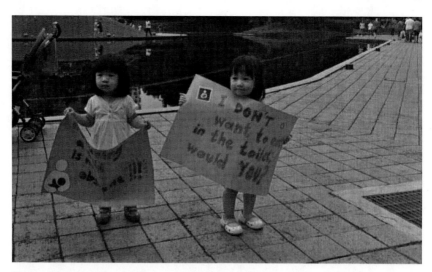

Figure 6.2. Malaysian children with World Breastfeeding Week posters, August 2011.

Chapter Seven

Mother Support Group Experience in Paraguay

Pushpa Panadam

INTRODUCTION

Paraguay is a landlocked country in the heart of South America with a Mediterranean-type climate and a total surface area of 406,752 km². It shares its borders with Bolivia in the north, Brazil in the northeast, and Argentina in the southeast and west (ENDSSR, 2008). The population of Paraguay is 6,381,940. It is unevenly distributed, with 59% in urban areas and 41% in rural areas (DGEEC, 2010a). The western region of Gran Chaco has 60% of the land area, but 97.3% of Paraguay's population lives in the eastern region (ENDSSR, 2008).

In 2009, with an annual birth rate of 154,000, the infant mortality rate was 19/1000 live births and the neonatal mortality rate was 12/1000 live births (UNICEF, 2011). Some of the causes of death are circumstances prior to birth, such as poverty, inadequate knowledge of childcare, limited access to healthcare services, inadequate attendance at the health services, deficiencies in the organization and functioning of the health services, lack in the quality of prenatal care, few medical/health consultations, and a late start to prenatal healthcare (Delgadillo, 2003). Other reasons for neonatal mortality are problems occurring during birth, infections, severe respiratory problems, and diarrhea (Organizacion Panamerica de la Salud, 2010). Breastfeeding immediately upon birth, exclusive breastfeeding for six months, and continuing breastfeeding with adequate, complementary feeding for two years and more would reduce and even prevent these deaths. Despite 94.2% breastfeeding initiation at birth, the present exclusive breastfeeding rate at six months is 24.4%.

Births in hospitals have increased in recent years to 84.6%, with 58.4% in public hospitals. Cesarean births have increased from 16.5% in 1998 to 33.1% in 2008. Home births, which occur mainly in rural areas and in the northern parts, have decreased to 11.5% (ENDSSR, 2008). Thus the role played in initiating breastfeeding with sufficient information to mothers in hospitals is really important. If pregnant women and mothers received the care stipulated under the Baby-Friendly Hospital Initiative (BFHI), exclusive breastfeeding would be high. However, factors that have made it difficult for hospitals accredited as Baby-Friendly Hospitals (BFH) to maintain their status or be accredited in the first place include:

- A lack of BFHI assessors, code monitoring, and continuous breastfeeding education
- A high turnover of hospital staff
- The weakness in implementing Step 10 of the BFHI, "Foster the establishment of breastfeeding support groups and refer mothers to them on discharge from the hospital or clinic."

The most effective type of mother support and mother support groups that must be available for pregnant women, mothers of newborns, breastfeeding mothers, and families are ones where the woman or mother feels she is being listened to, respected, and her feelings acknowledged, with opportunities to hear, share, and learn from other women and their experiences. The support group facilitators should believe in breastfeeding as the normal feeding method for infants and young children, have breastfeeding experience either of their own or from helping others, have communication skills and the ability to listen, and have an ability to provide the needed help and support. In Paraguay prior to 1983, this breastfeeding support for mothers was lacking.

In presenting the history of mother support in Paraguay, this chapter will address the following questions. Where do women go for information and support on breastfeeding during their pregnancies or after birth? What support groups are available for breastfeeding? Are they within easy access to the women and their family members? What problems do existing support groups face? If support groups are non-existent, insufficient, or not easily accessible, then what steps have been or are being taken to rectify this, either by the government or organizations working with mothers and babies?

HISTORY OF MOTHER SUPPORT IN PARAGUAY

Birth of La Leche League Paraguay

Bernadette Stäbler, a young German mother who had just arrived in Paraguay, was travelling through Yaguaron, a town 48 km from Asuncion, the capital. One of her first impressions of the country was the sight of a dead girl child, hardly two years old, in the arms of a person on the street. She was shocked and terribly heartbroken, as she was told that the child had died from diarrhea due to a lack of adequate milk. At that very moment, she was moved to establish a La Leche League (LLL) group in Paraguay.

Bernadette, who knew of LLL while in Germany, started her LLL Leader training immediately, even while she and her family were still living in a hotel, where they were for four months. She was accredited as a Leader in April 1983. (An LLL Leader is an experienced breastfeeding mother trained to give mother-to-mother support.) In September of that year, she founded La Liga de Leche Materna del Paraguay (LLLPy), conducting meetings for mothers from her home to help and support mothers to breastfeed their babies. Today there are 16 LLL Leaders in Paraguay—three are foreigners, two are married to Paraguayans.

EARLY LINK WITH THE HEALTH PROFESSIONALS

Mothers who attended Bernadette's monthly meetings were from her immediate neighborhood and other parts of Asuncion. Doctors and nurses who knew Bernadette and other mothers also came to these meetings which covered the four topics of the LLL "series" meetings—preparation during pregnancy, birth, breastfeeding, and gradual weaning with love. The meetings dealt with myths, including beliefs that breastfeeding alters or destroys breasts, spoils the child, and only the poor breastfeed. Another expatriate, Brigetta, the wife of the then German ambassador, was one of the mothers at these meetings. Her example showed other mothers that when more educated persons from a wealthier background breastfeed their babies, it is because they are aware that breastfeeding is important. Although the meetings were for mothers, the presence of doctors—especially pediatricians—and nurses was important. In the days before the Internet, Bernadette hoped that these health professionals would act as multipliers, reaching out to mothers with the information on the LLL Paraguay (LLLPy) group.

Dr. Flaviano Ojeda Villalba, Department of Nutrition, Ministry of Public Health and Social Welfare (MSPBS), attended the support group meetings. He was responsible for statistics for the Pan American Health Organization and the World Health Organization (PAHO /WHO). The mortality rate increased exponentially as children started bottle-feeding, especially in the rural areas. After reading the available information and materials, Bernadette and the mothers of her group felt they should reach out to medical students in the National University of Asuncion (UNA), the only medical faculty in Paraguay, so she donated breastfeeding pamphlets and materials from LLL

Paraguay to Dr. Flaviano. It was hoped that these materials could be used at the University and expose students to the idea that breastfeeding is normal and beneficial. There was no direct contact between LLLPy and the University or its students.

An invitation to visit the hospital came from the late Florencia Silva de Arnold, head nurse from the Hospital Cruz Roja Paraguaya (Red Cross Paraguay), now known as Hospital Materno Infantil Reina Sofía de la Cruz Roja (HCR). The salaries of the staff are paid by the MSPBS. Florencia was worried about bottle-feeding among the poor mothers in the maternity ward. These mothers thought that bottle-feeding showed others they could afford formula. It was, however, a different story when they went home, as they could not afford formula on a low income. Bernadette and Dorothy, experienced breastfeeding mothers, showed nurses how to help new mothers breastfeed. With Adriana, fluent in Paraguay's second official language—Guarani—they visited mothers in the maternity ward of HCR every week to help each mother with breastfeeding and bonding with her baby. They did not, however, start a support group at the hospital.

These early LLLPy mothers not only supported the mothers at the hospital, but also donated breastmilk for the orphans. Mothers who were breastfeeding exclusively upon leaving the hospital received a diploma (Figures 7.1, 7.2, 7.3), as Bernadette had observed that diplomas played a very important role in the Paraguayan culture. The diplomas were sponsored by LLLPy and HCR, and contained breastfeeding information and Frequently Asked Questions. Soon 100% of the mothers received these diplomas when they were discharged from the hospital. Visits to help mothers in the maternity ward at HCR were possible because Florencia (who died in 2011) and Dr. Claudio di Martino, a pediatrician, knew Bernadette, knew her work, and had asked her for help (B. Stäbler, personal communication, 2011).

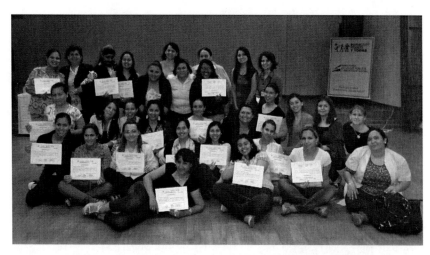

Figure 7.1. Trainee tutors with their certificates after the Ministry of Health course on Red Amamanta Paraguay. (See p. 98) Photo by Pushpa Panadam.

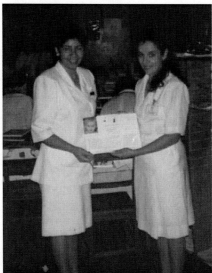

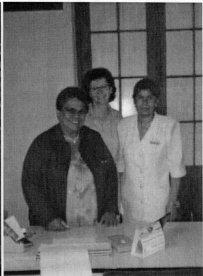

Figure 7.2. Nurses at Hospital Cruz Roja with the certificates provided by La Leche League of Paraguay in the 1980s for mothers who were exclusively breastfeeding when they left the hospital. Photo by Bernadette Stäbler.

Figure 7.3. At Hospital Cruz Rojas, Paraguay. Left to right: The late Florencia Silva de Arnold (head nurse), Bernadette Stäbler (LLL), and Arsenia Gonzáles (nurse). Photo by Bernadette Stäbler.

Evolution of LLL Support Groups

The first group of LLL Leaders accredited in early 1988, Americans Alba Valdovinos, Dorothy de Burt, and Paraguayan Lidia de Verón (Lily), led the series meetings alternatively in their homes after Bernadette left for Germany in late 1987. In 1991, three more Leaders were accredited. The meetings were rotated every four months in the Leaders' homes to allow mothers from other areas to have access to information and support. Meetings were held on different days of the month, usually weekdays, from 3:00 p.m. to 5:00 p.m. or 5:00 p.m. to 7:00 p.m. The earlier times attracted stay-at-home mothers and those who worked half days or had flexible working hours. However, mothers who worked full time or lived very far from the meeting place could not attend these meetings. Meeting times also depended on the host Leader and her family's needs.

In 1997, three permanent groups were formed, two in Asuncion and one in Fernando de la Mora. Mothers now had access to support group meetings all year around and more if they wanted. When the meeting group became too large for homes (15 to 20 mothers), Leaders organized meetings at a cooperative hall or a community center nearby. Having permanent meetings at one particular place is ideal for the host Leader with small children, and it is also good if mothers know with certainty the place, date, and time of the monthly support group meetings. Today there are two LLL monthly support groups in Leaders' homes in Paraguay: Lily's group in Asuncion and Elizabeth's in Fernando de la Mora. Another Leader, Cyntia, and I facilitate two mother support groups every month in HCR. Leaders provide face-to-face counseling, home visits, and telephone help; support family members, friends, and workmates; and give talks at schools, university, hospitals, and even at conferences (deVerón, 2003-2004).

Through the years Lily has tried to adapt the meeting times to suit the needs of younger mothers. She has held monthly Saturday evening meetings, so young mothers who are working or studying, or both, could come. As the babies of the group grew, mothers prioritized Saturday evenings for family commitments. So Lily now holds her evening meetings on weekdays (L. Gonzalez de Verón, P. Peña, E. Gavilan, & C. Leon, personal communication, 2011).

Challenges Faced When Leaders Facilitate Community Support Groups

Mothers, fathers, families, and the medical profession need to know that there are breastfeeding support groups that hold meetings once a month. They need to be aware of where, when, and how long these meetings take place. Meeting information must reach not only women, mothers, and families, but also the health service. Leaders spend time and money making phone calls, sending messages, and even sending emails informing friends and family of the meetings. This is money unaccounted for and comes out of the family budget.

Advertising meetings in newspapers is expensive. Most families do not buy newspapers every day, and the better newspapers are expensive for low-income families. Those families with Internet access (13.8%) (DGEEC, 2010b) read news online and perhaps only the sections that interest them.

For families from middle and upper classes or those with easy access to the Internet at home or in the workplace, meeting information, contact numbers, or email addresses of Leaders can be obtained easily. Having a network, like the LLL Spanish Leaders electronic mailing list, also helps as mothers learn of meetings and Leader contacts through Leaders from other parts of the world. Younger Leaders have set up a Facebook page for LLLPy. Mothers have also started to contact Leaders, having accessed phone numbers through the LLLI website (www.llli.org). However, the problem still remains for those who do not have access to Internet or computers to know that there is help available for breastfeeding problems.

Not knowing how many women, mothers, and family members will attend the meeting is a problem for Leaders planning meetings at home. Should they plan for many or only for a few, especially when it comes to chairs, food, etc.? Even though no one may show up, the Leader has to be prepared all the same. Leaders also have to cope with latecomers in support groups. The invitees may show up late for monthly meetings and stay later. This impinges on the Leaders' family time, especially with husbands and children coming back from work or school (P. Peña, C. Leon, E. Gavilan, & A. Maciel, personal communication, 2011). Being late for meetings, informal gatherings, birthday parties, and family meetings is part of the Paraguayan Culture. *Hora Paraguay*, or the "Paraguayan hour," can be anywhere from half an hour to more than an hour. Interestingly enough, this Hora Paraguay does not extend to schools, official meetings, or football games!

Sometimes mothers may not realize the importance of breastfeeding, but come to the meetings on the recommendation of their pro-breastfeeding doctors. These concerned doctors ask the Leaders to call these mothers, hoping that attending the meetings might help the new mother make an attempt at breastfeeding.

In the rural towns, mothers may be reluctant to seek a stranger's help in breastfeeding. Many mothers do not want to go to a place or home where they do not know anyone (L. Bowen, personal communication, 2011). Culturally, people are not used to going to a stranger's home where they will meet new people and be expected to share openly or ask questions. They are more used to passive listening, although once they are familiar with the other mothers, they do open up. Yet Paraguayans are used to meetings at schools, churches, and clubs they belong to.

There may be other practical difficulties. Leaders lend breastfeeding books to pregnant women and mothers to read and check on the women's progress, but sometimes books are not returned. Correct information on breastfeeding is often not available to mothers unless they receive it at the hospitals that actively promote breastfeeding, or they are directed to existing support groups or trained breastfeeding counselors. Support groups continue to change constantly as babies grow older and stop breastfeeding, and their mothers stop coming. Unless there are new mothers continuing to come, a group might stop growing and come to a standstill.

COMMUNITY OUTREACH

LLLPy Leaders, since the time of Bernadette, have often reached out to needy women and mothers beyond support groups. Their community outreach has taken different forms, for instance, in hospitals, in marginal communities, and in homes for abandoned teenagers.

Casa Rosa Maria

LLL Leader, Lily, a psychologist by profession, apart from facilitating a monthly support group in her house, also provides weekly support for pregnant adolescents and teen mothers at Casa Rosa Maria, Asuncion. The home's regulations allow the girls to stay for two months after the baby is born. Some girls, however, stay on longer, for up to a year until proper homes where they can live and work are found for them. There are usually about six to eight girls from 12 to 20 years old. The themes discussed during the meetings are flexible. Questions asked by the girls after overcoming their shyness mainly relate to changes occurring in their bodies and about caring for their babies. The teen mothers breastfeed their babies exclusively for the time they are at the home, and for the first six months if they stay on beyond the stipulated two months (L. Gonzalez de Verón, personal communication, 2011).

Abasto—Central Market

Elizabeth started childcare courses for parents in the Municipality Central Market, Abasto, in Asuncion. The turnout, however, was disappointing.

She feels that in order to attract families to support meetings and courses related to childcare, one must include crafts or learning a skill that would enable them to earn a living or improve their economic situation (E. Gavilan, personal communication, 2011).

Parhupar

The cesarean birth rate is on the rise in Paraguay. In 1998, 16.5% of all births were cesarean; in 2004, 26.9%; and by 2008, it had climbed to 33.1% (ENDSSR, 2008, p. 239). Concerned about the sexual and reproductive health of Paraguayan women and this high cesarean rate, some professional women, including a few LLL Leaders, founded *Parhupar* (*Parto Humanizado Paraguay*) in 2003. The main objective of Parhupar is to investigate, develop, and implement projects, programs, and actions that promote integrated care for the mother, young child, and family.

Early in 2005, Parhupar worked on a project, *School for Mothers and Future Mothers*, in Pelopincho, a marginalized community in the vicinity of HCR. Mother support group methodologies were used throughout the project, empowering women, providing them with tools to support other women and mothers in their community. Project mothers breastfed their babies exclusively and continued breastfeeding for more than a year.

In May 2007 under the Ministry sponsorship, Parhupar trained some of the women from this community and two men as peer counselors. Although some of these counselors indicated an interest in starting a group, it is difficult unless these volunteers receive economic support or other benefits, as this is usual in projects carried out in their communities by various organizations. Projects and programs in Pelopincho were conducted mainly in Spanish. However, the Jopará and Guarani languages were often used by the participants.

Guarani—The Other Official Language of Paraguay

The population of Paraguay is bilingual, which makes the country unique in South America. Guarani is the other official language in Paraguay, as guaranteed by the 1992 National Constitution of Paraguay. The language issue may pose a barrier in providing information and support to breastfeeding mothers. According to the 2002 census, 40% of the population spoke Jopará, a mixture of Spanish and Guarani. Guarani is the most frequently spoken language at home (59%), followed by Spanish (35.8%), and others (5%) (ENDSSR, 2008, p. 57). Despite the introduction of bilingual education in 1998, there are Spanish-speaking adults who may not have studied Guarani in schools nor been exposed to the language in their daily lives.

Three LLLPy Leaders are fluent in Guarani and are comfortable working with mothers in this language. Leaders who understand, but are not fluent, use Jopará, which is useful when carrying out workshops on peer counseling in rural regions. The ability to understand and speak Guarani fluently helps break barriers and creates a warmer atmosphere, enabling them to communicate more openly about breastfeeding.

There is no language issue for Leaders who do not understand or speak Guarani as the mothers who call, email, or attend LLLPy breastfeeding support groups are Spanish-speaking, usually from middle or upper class families and urban centers. Most Guarani speakers in urban areas are bilingual in Spanish and Guarani. In the socioeconomic breakdown, Guarani is commonly spoken by 76.5% of the population in extreme poverty. Problems may arise when someone tries to help mothers in Guarani if Guarani is not her mother tongue. This is the case of the indigenous population in Paraguay who are educated in one of the indigenous languages and Spanish.

Fluency in Guarani is an advantage for health personnel working in rural communities, but knowing Guarani does not guarantee that mothers will receive the help they need. Breastfeeding helpers and health workers need to learn not only how to incorporate breastfeeding information that is correct and up-to-date, but also be skillful in communication tools to support the families, promoting breastfeeding more effectively in the community. Words are not necessary when actions convey messages more convincingly.

The Ministry of Public Health and Social Welfare (MSPBS) in Paraguay does not provide printed materials in Guarani because the Guarani-speaking population is not Guarani literate. Written Guarani differs from the Guarani commonly spoken. However, LLL Leader Alicia Villalba has translated breastfeeding materials into Guarani for use in her University classes where she teaches students of health science and nursing (LLL Leaders: P. Peña, L. Bowen, N. Vega, A. Fracchia, M. Lopez, G. Ramirez, P. Gimenez, E. Gavilan, L. Gonzalez, C. Leon, L. Baez de Ibarra, A. Villalba, M. de Cáceres, A. Maciel, S. Olmedo, personal communication, 2011; Nurse S. Recalde, personal communication, 2011).

PEER COUNSELORS

In 2007-2008 the MSPBS was concerned with the lack of support groups in hospitals and in the community, and launched peer counselor training in two urban hospitals for recertifying as BFH, and in seven districts in the Department of Caaguazu and in Pelopincho where LLLPy and Parhupar participated (S. Recalde, personal communication, 2011). The Ministry, UNICEF, and LLLPy developed breastfeeding cloth posters adapted from cloth posters from LLL Guatemala and LLL Bolivia for this project. The cloth posters overcome language issues and the need for technology and come with a beautiful backpack for easy carrying. Peer counselors within Asuncion and other regions received these bag packs for their support work with mothers in their communities.

The main obstacle in this project was a lack of follow-up after the peer counselors were trained because of a lack of funding. Without follow-up and monitoring, peer counselors lose interest and the project fails in achieving its target—establishing mother support groups in different communities and regions country-wide, so mothers receive correct information and support on breastfeeding.

BABY-FRIENDLY HOSPITALS

There are currently 18 Baby-Friendly Hospitals (BFH) in Paraguay. It began with a MSPBS resolution creating an Executive Committee for Breastfeeding Promotion on July 2, 1991, renamed *Comisión Nacional de Fomento de la Lactancia Materna* (COFOLAM) on July 28, 1993. Responsible for certifying hospitals for the BFHI, COFOLAM consisted of teaching staff from pediatrics, doctors, nurses, and heads of departments of pediatrics and obstetrics of HCR and Hospital de Clinicas (Teaching hospital, Medical Faculty of UNA), MSPBS, and Instituto Prevision Social (IPS). La Leche League of Paraguay helped in the formation of support groups for the initiative. (Delgadillo, 2002).

Dr. Marta Gamarra of COFOLAM explained that although LLLPy helped in Step 10 with support groups and training community peer counselors for five hospitals in Asuncion, most of them are tertiary care or referral hospitals and some are also teaching hospitals. The women and mothers come to the hospitals for birth and are not necessarily from the local communities. Their prenatal and postnatal care is often carried out at the healthcare centers or other hospitals in their towns. Upon discharge from the hospital, they return to their communities, sometimes from towns and areas that are two, three, or even more hours away. Because the same support was not possible outside Asuncion, Step 10 was adapted to training health staff, nurses, and doctors in breastfeeding management to provide breastfeeding support to mothers while in these hospitals (M. Gamarra, personal communication, 2011).

Melania Gonzales, a nurse in HCR involved in BFHI, had her baby during the BFHI process, and the support she received helped her exclusively breastfeed her baby. This personal experience strengthened her conviction to help mothers succeed in their experience to this day. She encouraged pharmacies close to the hospital not to sell formulas and pacifiers and invited pharmacy staff to the talks held at the hospital. This was important as MSPBS monitored these places during the BFHI assessment process (M. Gonzales, personal communication, 2011).

Support Groups at Hospitals

Obstacles faced with earlier support groups in the hospitals were lack of support from the staff and a proper meeting place. Meetings took place in passageways and corridors (L. Gonzalez de Veron, P. Peña, personal communication, 2011). When mothers leave these BFHI hospitals, they should know of the availability of mother support groups. An evaluation of the BFHs in Paraguay in 2000/2001 by MSPBS and UNICEF found this terribly lacking. COFOLAM practically ceased to exist after this evaluation process. Today three of the BFHs and one private hospital in Asuncion have mother support groups or have started them.

Hospital Cruz Roja

The contact between LLLPy and HCR has continued since the time of Bernadette with few interruptions. Leaders help mothers in the maternity ward, plan World Breastfeeding Week (WBW) meetings, actively participate in WBW events, and give talks on Mother Support at training workshops for the health staff. HCR today has two monthly mother support groups facilitated by two Leaders.

In 2000 some of the medical staff began to coordinate HCR's Breastfeeding Committee (the Committee) (M. Parada de Ramirez, personal communication, 2011). This support made possible regular LLLPy Leader involvement in support group work at HCR, with weekly mother support groups in the pediatric department's waiting room.

The Committee includes representatives from all sections of the hospital working directly with mothers and babies: medical doctors (pediatricians and gynecologists/obstetricians), nurses, and psychologists, etc. The

Committee meets once or twice a month to ensure breastfeeding protection, promotion, and support on every level, including yearly training workshops for hospital residents and new staff, as well as the coordination of WBW activities with organizations working with mothers and babies.

Dr. Mireya Ramirez, who is at HCR three times a week monitoring breastfeeding efforts, invited Pushpa to a breastfeeding committee meeting. LLL Leaders often participate in WBW planning meetings held at HCR from March of each year. Yet the first time someone who was not a hospital staff member attended the committee's meeting to discuss internal issues, some people felt unduly uncomfortable. Acceptance came rapidly as mother support with volunteer help was indispensable, as was the sharing of consistent breastfeeding resources and information.

The idea to start a monthly mother support group, or club, was immediately welcomed. A place, a day, and a time was fixed, and the health staff in the pediatric department was informed of the club meetings in July 2007. The meetings are held at a consultation room in the pediatric department, from 8:30 a.m. to 10:00 a.m. to entice mothers and families from the waiting room to the meeting. Mothers initially feared losing their turns. It was resolved by talking to the doctors, nurses, and volunteers who called mothers during the meeting. Mothers are encouraged to come for the next consultation at a time when support group meetings are held to avoid too many trips to the hospital, as some of them travel from afar by bus.

The mother support group is also a learning experience for doctors, nurses, and Cruz Roja volunteers. They are used to giving breastfeeding talks during prenatal care and in maternity wards, with talks sometimes a little too technical, standing facing the mothers and families. In the club they respect each mother, listen to her experience, and do not give lectures. They sit and share their own personal experiences as mothers, grandmothers, and aunts. Mothers or pregnant women attending the meetings are those who had their babies there or come for antenatal or postnatal care. These mothers are usually not from nearby communities or even from Asuncion.

When the club first started, mothers directed their questions more to the doctors instead of sharing their experiences or voicing their doubts to the group in general. However, over the last four years, this scenario has changed. The doctors share their experiences as working mothers, as supportive grandmothers to their daughters and daughters-in-law, and even how they support their domestic help at home with breastfeeding (Figure 7.4).

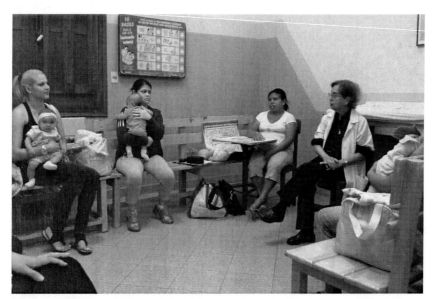

Figure 7.4. Mother support group in Paraguay. Cyntia Ortiz, a peer counselor from the Pelopincho community, is second from right (without a baby). Dr. Mireya is next to her. Photo by Pushpa Panadam.

A second mother's club for pregnant teens, women, and young mothers was started in May 2009 in the Adolescent Department. This group, facilitated by the same two Leaders, Dr. Mireya and Dr. Amanda Peña, meets monthly. The women who come to this meeting are usually first-time young pregnant women, teenagers from 14 years onwards, and Dr. Andres Gubetich from Hogar Maternal, who belongs to Cruz Roja Paraguaya (Paraguay Red Cross). Since the gynecological office is also in this section of the hospital, non-pregnant or women in the pre-menopausal stage are invited to share their experiences and learn more about breastfeeding support.

Maintaining HCR Mother Support Groups

Work related to mother support groups includes providing healthy snacks to mothers and families; informing the professional and non-professional staff of the meeting dates; and posting meeting and breastfeeding information on boards at the hospital entrance, prenatal area, maternity ward, the NICU, mother's shelter (for babies in NICU), and the pediatric department. Breastfeeding photos printed by the library assistant and important breastfeeding phrases from the Committee appear on the information boards and in the consultation room. These boards are kept current, which is a challenge because volunteers are not regulars at the hospital. Nurses in charge have to be reminded quite often because of their work overload.

At present the hospital receives fewer families from very low socio-economic background as compared to before and takes in more paying patients. Mothers with healthy babies may be reluctant to attend meetings unless they are there for consultation, especially during certain epidemic periods. Parents of sick babies often do not participate in the meetings.

Volunteers or Dr. Mireya collect data on where the baby was born or will be born (for pregnant women), type of birth, when the baby was first put the breast, and whether babies receive anything other than breastmilk. Problems faced by mothers while hospitalized for birth or when a baby is in the NICU are noted. Mothers are asked if they received breastfeeding information during prenatal care, how they were treated by hospital staff, when babies were put to the breast after birth, where the baby is placed during transfer from labor room to maternity ward (on mother's chest or between her legs), and other questions. Mothers whose babies are in intensive care and fed breastmilk via cups by nurses may return home without being shown how to do it themselves. The information gathered is then discussed at the committee level on how to improve hospital practices.

Every year the clubs celebrate their anniversary months, WBW, and end of the year festival. Families and hospital staff, including the heads of the neonatology unit and hospital, participate equally in these events. The parties are celebrated with cakes, treats, gifts, and a slideshow of photos taken during the year.

On July 5, 2011, we celebrated the fourth year of HCR Mother's Club. Despite a bus strike and really cold weather, there were five mothers with their babies, three pregnant women, a grandmother, a Cruz Roja volunteer, three pediatricians, and two LLL Leaders. One of the mothers came with her almost three-year-old, especially to share her experience on breastfeeding beyond two years. One pediatrician participated for the first time at the club. She enthusiastically shared her personal experience as a mother of three boys and how difficult it was as a medical resident to breastfeed her oldest son. But today she supports her niece to nurse beyond three years (P. Panadam, personal communication, 5 July 2011).

PROBLEMS FACED BY MOTHERS

The problems mothers face include sore nipples, cracked nipples, no milk, insufficient milk, a baby who wants to feed often, or a baby who is "hungry." These worries arise from insufficient or incorrect information received during prenatal care and lack of sufficient help regarding effective positioning and latching during the 24 to 48 hours the mother is in the hospital. First time mothers are usually not certain of reading infant cues, and may not know babies need to breastfeed often, how to check if the baby is getting enough milk, or how their milk supply can be increased.

Support From the Community Peer Counselors

Because of the closeness of the Pelopincho community to HCR, some peer counselors trained by Parhupar come when asked to support ongoing groups at the hospitals. Since it is voluntary work, hospitals must be within walking distance. These women must also be available to attend and help at these meetings. Many of them, once trained, are more confident and able to find employment faster. So even if they are willing to help or run a group, they are unable to do so unless there is some kind of economic benefit.

Hospital Barrio Obrero

The author was a stay-at-home mother and LLL Leader, whose children's after school activities began to clash with the 3:00-5:00 p.m. monthly LLL meetings. Wanting to continue helping mothers and babies, from August 2001 until 2007, I volunteered weekly at Hospital Barrio Obrero (HBO), a BFH facility two blocks from my house. Some doctors and nurses were interested and supported my breastfeeding work and have helped in organizing WBW activities since 2002.

When HCR started its support group in 2007, it was easier to facilitate the monthly groups there with support from the committee. Learning that changes must occur not only with mother and baby, but also with the staff, I kept in touch with them, the head nurses, and some of the doctors, providing information on WBW and breastfeeding. When a need arose for a Breastfeeding Management workshop, Parhupar, with funding from Latchon, ran an 18-hour course in 2009 for the staff and nursing students. Dr. Mireya of HCR was one of the facilitators for the workshop.

On April 6, 2011, a support group was started with Nurse Sonia, head nurse of the maternity section of HBO, for mothers of babies in intensive care. These mothers live in a shelter within the hospital. They are interested in learning how to hand express, store their breastmilk, and how to breastfeed when their babies are well. Sonia learned that a support group works best when mothers introduce themselves and give a brief introduction into their lives. Further barriers were broken when she shared her experiences and asked what problems they faced. Mothers worried about restricted time with their babies in the Neonatal Care Unit (NCU) and also that they experienced losing their expressed milk stored there, for instance, if it was used by other mothers. Relying on the head nurse to run the support group is difficult due to her workload.

In August 2011, with WBW events at both the hospital and participation in the *Feria de Lactancia Materna* (Breastfeeding Fair) organized by HCR in the city center, interest in mother support and breastfeeding has increased. The public health section of HBO has started organizing mother support group meetings on a weekly basis.

Hospital Materno Infantil Fernando de la Mora

In October 2010, LLL Leaders Elizabeth and Avelina Macieal (Lika) started a support group at Hospital Materno Infantil Fernando de la Mora, in the town where they both live (E. Gavilan, A. Maciel, personal communication, 2011). The Leaders were supported by a nurse and two doctors. However, from January to March, 2011, the dengue epidemic in the country resulted in a lack of meeting space for the group as human resources were diverted to cope with the crisis.

Hospital Bautista

Hospital Bautista, a private hospital in Asuncion (not BFHI-accredited), has had a support group for parents for more than 20 years, started by Jane Jones, a missionary from the USA. According to Nurse Elsa Velazquez (personal communication, 2011), who coordinates and facilitates the group, meeting preparations often take time. Representatives of a private company helped make 50 phone calls per meeting to invite families and help during the meetings, but no longer. Usually 10 to 12 mothers, who typically have given birth at the hospital or are friends of the families, would come. The mother support group is free, although Elsa also runs a paying course for parents. Elsa, who also teaches nursing students at the Universidad Centro Medico Bautista, said that breastfeeding is part of its course for students (personal communication).

Hospital Materno Infantil San Pablo

The first human milk bank (HMB) in Paraguay in Hospital San Pablo (HBM HSP) was inaugurated in April 2010, after a course on processing and quality control in human milk banks was conducted by Red Iberoamericano. The percentages of premature and low birthweight babies in the hospital who received only human milk from the bank were 88% in January and 92.8% in February. The percentage of mothers who received breastfeeding counseling increased from 75% in January to 80% in

February 2011. When the milk bank celebrated its first anniversary, donor mothers and their children came from different parts of the country and were honored with certificates, gifts, and a lovely tea, which included a cake with breastfeeding mothers on it (Figure 7.5).

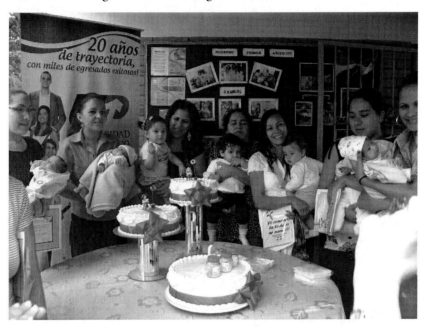

Figure 7.5. First anniversary celebration of the Human Milk Bank in Hospital San Pablo. (The banner celebrates 20 years since the founding of the Universidad del Pacifico, one of the sponsors of the milk bank.)

The staff at the HMB HSP (milk bank) held their first monthly support group on July 28, 2011. Dr. Marta Herrera, HMB director, invited health staff, educators, mothers from the community, and those with hospitalized babies. Dr. Mireya and I were invited to facilitate the group meeting, using the small office of the HMB. Individual breastfeeding experiences were shared, including by the staff. One mother's quadruplets were in the NICU. One baby died, but the remaining three received banked human milk and their mother's expressed milk. Dr. Mireya explained to the staff that it was important to work and support the volunteers (or peer counselor/LLL Leader). "We need to bring ourselves to the level of the mothers, share our experiences from that human angle," she said.

Hospital San Pablo is a BFH-accredited facility, yet there was no mother support group in the hospital or in the communities close by. Ida Pereira, a nurse at HSP since becoming a BFH, said starting a mother support group has been difficult, although there is a *Club de Lactante* (breastfeeding club).

According to Dr. Marta Herrera, due to the dengue epidemic earlier this year, the club has been suspended.

The HMB helps mothers whose babies are hospitalized, through counseling and teaching how to hand express. This accounts for about 75% of their work. The rest includes pasteurizing the collected or donated milk, preparing portions for the day, and promoting the collecting post for breastmilk (like HCR, HBO) for the milk bank. Mothers initially express breastmilk for their own babies. They are discharged when their babies begin to breastfeed. It is these mothers, now confident in their breastfeeding ability, who become breastmilk donors. However, this being a referral hospital, most mothers come from other areas. HMB goes to the mothers' individual homes and hospitals in other towns to collect the donated milk (M. Herrera, personal communication, 2011).

A regular mother support group with mothers from the community would help the milk bank as their donors would be closer, and time and money would be saved on trips to far-off places. Since the July mother support group meeting, the HMB has actively participated in World Breastfeeding Week activities organized within the hospital and by HCR in the Breastfeeding Fair. The second support group meeting was held in early September with more mothers from the community.

Unidad de Salud de la Familia

Unidads de Salud de la Familia (USF), or Family Health Units, provide free primary healthcare directly to the people in the community. They are small multi-professional, functional units run by doctors, nurses, administrators, and others. They may be the answer to exclusive breastfeeding and breastfeeding with adequate and complementary feeding for two years and beyond for mothers in the communities who do not have access to the referral hospitals and BFHI.

The September 29, 2011, edition of *Ultima Hora* reported the Vice Health Minister's statement that 503 USFs have been installed in 18 sanitary regions this year, with an additional 200 planned. More than two million people, who before were out of the health system because no hospitals were available, will benefit. The installation of these Units is a priority for MSPBS and the Secretariat for Social Action, especially in the poorest zones. Each Unit team includes community health promoters from the local community.

The USFs are at the heart of the community. The team knows each and everyone in the community personally. Each USF is responsible for about 3,500-4,000 people. The health or community workers go from house to house and provide help and information to pregnant women, as well as mothers of newborns and young children. They also provide training for the team and support meetings for families are held weekly. Although women have their babies at the hospitals, they come to the USF for their continued postnatal appointments.

Red Amamanta Paraguay

A five-day, 40-hour training for 28 tutors to address breastfeeding and complementary feeding in primary care at the Unidad Salud de la Familia (USF) took place in September 2011. The trainees ran a six-hour workshop in four USFs in poor communities and launched Red Amamanta Paraguay. The project, sponsored by the MSPBS and UNICEF, is modeled after Red Amamanta Brasil. Red Amamanta Paraguay consists of a strategy based on constructing a new paradigm for teaching breastfeeding, recognizing each participant's background knowledge, and respecting his/her perceptions of it. The two main aspects of Red Amamanta are its permanent or continuous education and Critical Reflexive Education.

Red Amamanta Paraguay plans to work through the USFs to provide breastfeeding support to mothers as health promoters visit pregnant women, mothers of newborns, and babies in their houses. Some of the units have started breastfeeding support groups. The health and community workers in USFs must be trained to facilitate mother support groups and also be skillful in breastfeeding management and communication. As tutors of Red Amamanta Paraguay, they will be expected to run workshops, training the USF team to work in a supportive way with families and to listen to their stories and their experiences.

CONCLUSION

Breastfeeding mother support today is provided by LLL Leaders on a monthly basis in their homes and at some hospitals, along with telephone help, home visits, email, and Facebook. Mothers and families, however, must be able to access information about the meetings and available help. The challenge is in getting this information to them prior to and after birth and to the health professionals.

Mother support groups succeed at hospitals with a supportive breastfeeding committee. Mothers and pregnant women not only receive correct information and help, but also receive continued support through pregnancies, birth, and the postnatal period.

Families in rural regions and marginal communities may get the breastfeeding support they require at USFs. Mother support groups at USFs must be facilitated by health professionals and community leaders proficient in Guarani who are trained in basic breastfeeding management and communication skills, with ongoing trainings to keep them up-to-date with breastfeeding information.

Mother support group meetings should be held in a permanent place if possible and information made available through television (reaching 87.7% of the population), radio, and mobile phones (reaching 85.1%) (DGEEC, 2010b).

Support for those *providing* support is also important. A network must be built within the hospitals, among hospitals and healthcare systems, with qualified breastfeeding counselors, like LLL Leaders, and with nursing and medical professionals. Providing and exchanging current information to professionals is an important step in building this informal network of breastfeeding supporters.

Chapter Eight

Peer Counseling for Increasing Exclusive Breastfeeding: Experiences from Bangladesh

Rukhsana Haider, MD, MSc, PhD, IBCLC

INTRODUCTION

The People's Republic of Bangladesh is a small, but thickly populated country (approx. 159 million in 147,570 sq. km), surrounded by India on three sides, Myanmar along the southeast border, and the Bay of Bengal in the south. The country has mainly flat alluvial plains with low hills in the northeast and southeast, and the climate is semitropical, with monsoons. About three-fourths of the population is rural, but rural-urban migration is leading to a rapid increase in the urban population, mainly the poor.

Although breastfeeding is still common in the first two years, both the breastfeeding and complementary feeding practices in the country are far from satisfactory. This contributes to the high child malnutrition rates, with about 40% of children below five years of age malnourished, as reported in the national Bangladesh Demographic Health Surveys (BDHS) conducted during the last fifteen years (Mitra, Ali, Islam, Cross, & Saha, 1994; Mitra, Al-Sabir, Cross & Jamil, 1997; National Institute of Population Research and Training, 2001, 2005, 2009). Noting the high child malnutrition rates, a Campaign for the Protection, Promotion, and Support for Breastfeeding (CPPBF) was initiated nationally in 1989, mainly by pediatricians, nutritionists, program staff working in child health programs, and other concerned individuals and organizations. The campaign was supported by the United Nations Children's Fund (UNICEF) and the World Health Organization (WHO/UNICEF, 1989). After launching the Baby-Friendly Hospital Initiative (BFHI) by UNICEF and WHO in 1991, further impetus was given to the Breastfeeding Campaign, and training of maternity health facility staff, as per global recommendations, became a priority. From the International Centre for Diarrheal Disease and Research, Bangladesh (ICDDR,B), I was deputed first to Campaign for the

Protection, Promotion, and Support for Breastfeeding (which was funded mainly by UNICEF), and then to UNICEF to help establish the BFHI, including supervision of training and implementation of the International Code of Marketing of Breastmilk Substitutes. The 40-hour breastfeeding counseling course (WHO, 1993) was field tested in Bangladesh, and my involvement with the training program increased over the following years, from conducting the first official national breastfeeding counseling course to many other courses conducted nationally and internationally.

Purpose

By the late 1990s, since the BFHI was a priority program of the Government of Bangladesh, training had been provided to staff in many maternity health facilities and hospitals certified as Baby-Friendly, but utilization of these facilities by pregnant women was extremely low. Only one-third of the pregnant women went for antenatal checks, and around 80% of the women gave birth to babies at home, attended mostly by unskilled birth attendants (Mitra et al., 1994). As these women were not getting the essential breastfeeding information, no significant changes could be reported in actual breastfeeding practices, particularly in exclusive breastfeeding. Peer counseling programs had been shown to be useful in increasing breastfeeding initiation and duration in other parts of the world (Kistin, Abramson, & Dublin, 1994; Alvarado et al., 1996; Leite et al., 1998), but had not been organized in Asia. This led us to study whether peer counseling would be effective in increasing and sustaining exclusive breastfeeding prevalence rates in selected areas of Bangladesh.

The peer counseling program described in this chapter is based in two locations: Anowara, a rural sub-district (*upazila*) of Chittagong division (south-east Bangladesh) and Badda in Dhaka (the capital of Bangladesh), which is an urban lower-middle-class community with pockets of slums. Although we are working to improve infant and young child feeding practices in totality, only experience from the breastfeeding component of the program will be described in this chapter (as the complementary feeding aspects are being presented elsewhere).

History

Working at the International Center for Diarrheal Disease, Bangladesh (ICDDR,B) hospital in Dhaka, it was quite noticeable to us over several years that the children being admitted with diarrhea were getting younger. Whereas in earlier years toddlers and young children came with diarrhea, they were being replaced by infants as young as a few weeks and even a few days old, basically because they were only partially breastfed. Even though some of these infants had been delivered at health facilities, their mothers had not received adequate breastfeeding information. There was no organized community-based support system in place to encourage and guide the mothers. Seeing this as a missed opportunity to inform and provide the required skills to mothers of young infants, the first counseling research project was undertaken in that diarrheal disease hospital, although there were arguments about its suitability as it was not a maternity facility. Breastfeeding counselors were recruited and trained using the WHO counseling course, and then mothers of admitted, partially breastfed infants below three months of age with diarrhea, but without other complications, were counseled to stop other milk and convert to exclusive breastfeeding (Haider et al., 1996). The results showed that 60% of mothers were exclusively breastfeeding at discharge (usually between three to five days) versus 6% of mothers in the control group who received only the usual health education messages. These figures had increased to 75% and 8% (p<0.001), respectively, when followed up at home two weeks later, after the babies' full recovery from diarrhea when oral rehydration solution was stopped.

Following these encouraging results and recognizing the limitations of counseling only those mothers who would bring their sick young infants to the hospital, the next step was to take preventive measures instead of waiting for the damage to occur and then to try to undo it. A community-based research project was thus undertaken in Badda, urban Dhaka. Women were selected to become peer counselors following certain selection criteria and trained using an adapted, simplified version of the 40-hour breastfeeding counseling course and other relevant materials (Haider, Kabir, Huttly, & Ashworth, 2002). Mothers were recruited in late pregnancy and received counseling. They were counseled again after delivery and monthly until their infants were five months old (as per the national recommendations during those days). Again the results were spectacular. While 70% of counseled mothers managed to exclusively breastfed their infants until they were five months old (as per national recommendations at that time), this was in striking contrast to only 6% of mothers who were not counseled (Haider, Ashworth, Kabir & Huttly, 2000). Subsequently, to determine whether peer counselors would also be useful in rural areas where mothers had extended families and support networks, the project was replicated in rural Anowara. Since six months of exclusive breastfeeding was being proposed globally, (WHO/UNICEF, 2003), we suggested that mothers practice accordingly. It was extremely gratifying that our suggestions were accepted, and again the results were extremely good as

89% and 85% of mothers breastfed exclusively for six months in the individually counseled and mixed groups, respectively (individual + group counseling) (Kabir & Haider, unpublished).

Even more encouraging was the fact that the community members really appreciated that their babies were growing well and staying healthy, without suffering from any major illness. Thus when the research ended, they requested that we should continue to guide and support the peer counselors, and this led us first to establish the Training and Assistance for Health & Nutrition (TAHN) Trust in 2000, and then the Foundation in 2008. Since then we have been very fortunate to have the goodwill and best wishes of communities in both the urban and rural sites and to be able to support the program from our own resources with donations from good friends. Other funding has included seed grants from the World Alliance for Breastfeeding Action (WABA) for World Breastfeeding Week activities and an 18-month grant from the World Bank (Nutrition Development Marketplace) which ended recently. Although initially there were 20 peer counselors in Badda and many batches trained over the years, only five are currently working there. Similarly in Anowara, the numbers have reduced from 20 to seven, primarily due to lack of external funds. Each peer counselor covers approximately 300 households and is responsible for 50-60 mothers at any one time. This includes pregnant women in the last trimester and infants below 12 months of age, so they can focus on exclusive breastfeeding and complementary feeding after six months.

Monitoring and Evaluation

Peer counselors maintain registers for obtaining information from mothers and use them to record their feeding practices. These registers are checked by program staff every month, and data is entered into computers, analyzed, and feedback is provided to the peer counselors. The program staff also carry out frequent supervision and monitoring visits, using checklists to ensure that the peer counselor's performance is satisfactory. However, to obtain an unbiased view of whether the program was still being effective in achieving and sustaining high exclusive breastfeeding prevalence, a rapid survey was undertaken in mid-2009. College girls were recruited and trained over four days to understand and use pre-tested questionnaires to interview mothers. Over 300 mothers were receiving peer counselor services at each site, so using sample size calculations that would detect a 30% difference from the national exclusive breastfeeding prevalence of 40%, every third mother was randomly selected for the interview. Thus 100 mothers were interviewed at the urban site and 100 mothers at the rural site. The survey showed that despite fewer monitoring visits (as compared to the research projects), the high exclusive breastfeeding rates continued to be maintained. These rapid survey results were used as a baseline when we undertook an intensified project in December 2009 (World Bank funded) to address infant and young child feeding practices, with increased emphasis on improving complementary feeding practices. This project ended in June 2011, but it has been most heartening to see that over the years, the exclusive breastfeeding prevalence rates continue to remain very high in the Foundation's areas, probably the highest in the country. Figure 8.1 shows this prevalence at different points in time over several years.

Figure 8.1. Prevalence of exclusive breastfeeding (EBF).

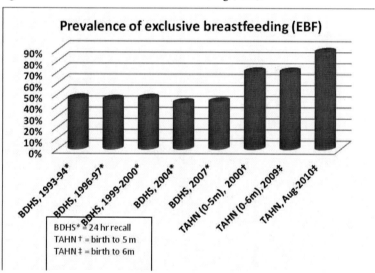

In addition to the monitoring visits, focus group discussions and in-depth interviews are conducted at frequent intervals to understand the perceptions of mothers and other family members. Some of the views expressed by mothers and fathers about the peer counseling services, as well as those of the peer counselors themselves, are highlighted below. Also included are a supervisor's views regarding the peer counseling program.

Pregnant mothers. In one focus group discussion, a pregnant mother said:

> This is my first baby. Whatever I know, I have learned from her (the TAHN Counselor)—about taking iron tablets, starting breastfeeding within one hour after baby is born, not giving sugar water, and then feeding only breastmilk for first six months of age, not even giving water.

Another pregnant mother said:

> I had heard some messages, but they were not very specific. For example, "eat more food" was a message, but how much more should be eaten was not mentioned. I learnt from the Counselor Apa (big sister) who visits that I should eat one fistful more of rice with curry at each meal, rest for two hours in the afternoon, also how to hold the baby for breastfeeding, etc.

MOTHERS WITH INFANTS UNDER SIX MONTHS. In another focus group discussion, the majority of mothers with infants under six months mentioned that they were feeding only breastmilk to their babies. They agreed with the mother who said, "I feed my baby only my milk and I have no problem in doing so." Another mother's story was:

> I have two children. My first child's age is seven years. I fed him only breastmilk till he was six months old. And I plan to feed only breastmilk till six months to my second child also. I learnt how to breastfeed from, Shirin (peer counselor) apa (sister), who worked in TAHN foundation earlier. Now sister, Rupa (current peer counselor in that area) comes to visit and explain how to feed the child breastmilk properly, how long I should feed my child breastmilk, etc. After delivery of this baby, I also started breastfeeding within one hour. I have learnt all this firstly from TAHN Foundation apas and now I also hear it on TV. I am also sharing the information with other mothers that feeding colostrum immediately after birth is necessary and good for the child's health.

Another mother said, "During these past five months I did not have to take my baby to the hospital even once. For a slight cold and fever, I bought some medicine from the pharmacy and he was okay." Asked if she thought the peer counselor's visit was useful, considering that she did not give any remedy, but only suggestions, one mother said, "Of course I have benefited from this sister's visit and I liked it. She gave good advice and said many useful things. This is more important." When mothers were asked if, after learning about these optimal child feeding practices, they would be able to apply this knowledge and these practices to their next children, or would they need further assistance, the mothers replied: "We will not forget what we have learnt. Obviously we will be able to feed our next children similarly, and we will also be able to advise others" (Figures 8.2, 8.3).

FATHERS. Fathers were very happy to be included in the discussions. One father said, "The peer counselor comes and advises my wife on how to feed the baby. She also shows how the baby is growing (on the growth card), which is very good. When she tells us that our baby is growing well, we feel happy." Another father said, "My younger baby was breastfed exclusively since aunt Hasina (peer counselor) advised my wife. I have seen with my own eyes the benefits of exclusive breastfeeding. This baby remained well, in contrast to my older child who was given other milk before six months, but often fell ill." He added, "Actually, no mother can breastfeed exclusively if she is not supported by her husband. I also used to encourage her to eat more so she could breastfeed more!"

PEER COUNSELORS. All the peer counselors said that they enjoyed the work. Those who were working outside their homes for the first time also said that they had not faced any problems. They had gained a lot of experience regarding breastfeeding (and complementary feeding), which they did not have, even though they were mothers themselves. They are now well recognized in the area and people stop to acknowledge them and talk to them whenever they see them. They have gained a lot of respect and feel happy and satisfied when mothers listen to their suggestions and practice accordingly, and babies grow well and remain healthy.

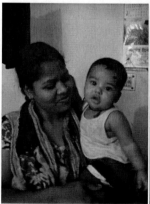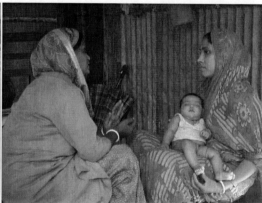

Figure 8.2. Urban mother, Momtaz, and her baby. Photo by Dr. Rukhsana Haider.

Figure 8.3. Mother support in Bangladesh. Photo by Dr. Rukhsana Haider.

A SUPERVISOR. A supervisor of the peer counselors said it was surprising that, although all the peer counselors were mothers who had breastfed their children, they did not have very clear ideas about what the national breastfeeding recommendations were. This needed to be explained to them, not only during training, but again during the field supervision and monitoring visits. Refresher training was also essential and effective, especially when role-plays and demonstrations were used. It was gratifying when mothers' breastfeeding practices were good, and they attributed this to the peer counselor, but frustrating when there were slips in their performance.

CHALLENGES

A question we face quite frequently is regarding the type of challenges we faced during implementation of the peer counseling program. Of course these were multiple when we first started the program. People were skeptical and questioned that—given that most women breastfeed—why women would need to be trained in something as natural as breastfeeding. The major challenge was to convince donors, and then community members, that even though Bangladesh is a country where breastfeeding is the tradition, the practices themselves are not optimal and that is one of the leading reasons for the high level of child malnutrition and frequent illness. The other challenges—and I do not like to call them barriers—are briefly listed below:

- Funding: This is the biggest challenge, as donors tend to go to big organizations, both for testing new ideas, and also to support longer-term programs.

- Urban problems: There are a lot of competing opportunities compared to those in rural areas. Everyone is on the lookout to earn more money, and attitudes also seem to have changed. Compared to a few years ago, women appear to be less motivated for community work.

- Staff availability and turnover: Here too, the main attraction is higher salaries. It is becoming increasingly difficult to find staff that are interested in community-based work and want to stay for several years with one organization.

- Product demand: As many non-government organizations distribute or provide free medicines or nutritional supplements, mothers ask for products (iron tablets, food supplementation packets, etc.).

- Income and education: Better educated families, or those with more income, prefer to go to doctors and follow their advice for adding breastmilk substitutes, even though it may be unnecessary.

- Many fathers who live away from their families like to bring breastmilk substitutes or fancy feeding bottles when they visit, especially if they come from the city or abroad, as these are thought to be prestigious and social status issues.

Conclusions and Scaling Up

The TAHN Foundation's peer counseling program in Bangladesh has been consistent in achieving high rates of exclusive breastfeeding and sustaining them over the years (Figure 8.1). The peer counselors' work is also appreciated, and they feel important and empowered, especially when they see that mothers follow their suggestions and their babies remain healthy and grow well. However, for their continued success, frequent monitoring and evaluation by program supervisors and feedback from them to the peer counselors is vital.

Breastfeeding counseling is now largely recognized as one of the effective interventions for improving child health (Bhutta et al., 2008), but in Bangladesh, as in many other countries, this knowledge has not really been applied. In mid 2009, findings from formative research conducted in rural Chittagong and urban Dhaka highlighted the fact that we are still lagging behind in many aspects, and programs that claim to promote breastfeeding definitely need to be strengthened further (Haider et al., 2010). Utilizing these research findings, the Alive & Thrive project of the Academy for Educational Development (USA) in their grant to the Bangladesh Rural Advancement Committee (BRAC - the world's largest NGO) has adopted the concept of peer counselors. TAHN shared the peer counseling training materials and monitoring checklists which were further adapted, and similar work is being done by a new cadre of full-time salaried staff, namely community-based women called "Infant and Young Child Feeding Promoters" or *Pushti Kormis*. These women work closely with community volunteers (*Shashthya Shebikas*) and their supervisors (*Shashthya Kormis*) to promote and support infant and young child feeding. In a recent AED presentation, it was reported that more than 5000 staff and volunteers have been trained to date (Sanghvi, unpublished).

In a research project conducted by ICDDR,B, community health workers and staff were trained by a TAHN breastfeeding supervisor and had good results in the early postnatal days (Mannan et al., 2008). ICDDR,B has now received funds for another peer counseling research project that will also look at the impact of the intervention on complementary feeding practices and on reducing growth stunting. TAHN staff will train the peer counselors and I will be closely involved with the implementation. Earlier, experiences from this peer-counseling model were utilized for developing a research project for counseling breastfeeding mothers with HIV in South Africa with impressive results (Bland, Rollins, Coovadia, Coutsoudis, & Newell, 2007).

So although we have not been able to provide peer counseling services directly in many parts of the country, our methods and results, as well as the trained staff, continue to contribute to and influence many infant and young child feeding projects and programs, both nationally and internationally. We hope that this will continue to expand in the coming years.

Chapter Nine

The Baby Café

Catherine Pardoe BSc, RN, IBCLC
Julie Williams MSc, RHV, IBCLC

INTRODUCTION

In the United Kingdom, only two thirds of babies are breastfed at birth, and just one in five is still receiving breastmilk at six months (Foster, 1995; NHS, 2000; Bolling et al., 2007). Most mothers report that they want to breastfeed their babies for longer. Community breastfeeding interventions in the United Kingdom are very fragmented, with some women accessing excellent care and others poorly supported (Langley, 1998; Frossell, 1998; Hoddinott & Roisin, 1999; National Breastfeeding Working Group, 1995).

It was within this climate that the first Baby Café drop-in support center was founded. A Baby Café breastfeeding center combines the expertise of other mums and skilled practitioners in a professional, but non-clinical, café-style environment. Ten years later, the number of Baby Cafés has increased ten-fold, with over 100 Baby Cafés mainly in the United Kingdom, but with a growing number in the USA, as well as in Singapore, China, and the Channel Islands.

PURPOSE AND PHILOSOPHY

From the beginning our highest intention was that all mothers—no matter what their ethnic, economic, or educational background—could access the information and help they need to breastfeed. In line with the Baby-Friendly Initiative, it was important to us that any community breastfeeding intervention would sit within a global, national, and local framework of excellent practice (WHO, 1981; UNICEF UK BFI, 2009; Department of Health, 2000).

Underpinning this philosophy was the desire to provide a service where we, as mothers ourselves, would feel comfortable, cared for, and valued. It was also a key requirement that we created a safe environment within a wider culture that often feels threatened by women's determination to overcome obstacles to their chosen method of parenting. Mothers are often isolated. Within a Baby Café drop-in, they can practice feeding. Antenatal mothers can chat with breastfeeding mothers and see babies being breastfed, perhaps for the first time, all in a non-threatening, comfortable setting.

> **MOTHER'S QUOTE:** "It's amazing how discreet you can be with practice—watching others helped [me] to overcome the initial anxieties of feeding in public. I'm sure this is why I breastfed for so long (eight months)."

In a Baby Café, breastfeeding is viewed as the expected method of feeding for a mother to nourish and nurture her child. The breastfeeding relationship at whatever stage is respected and protected (Figures 9.1, 9.2).

> **MOTHER'S QUOTE:** "The support and care that I received gave me the confidence to continue breastfeeding through a very painful time...."

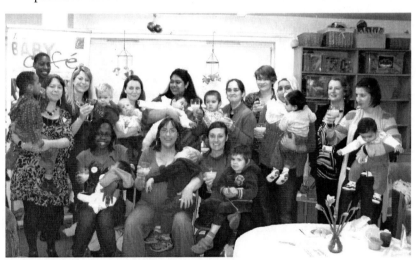

Figure 9.1. The Purley Baby Café in the United Kingdom.

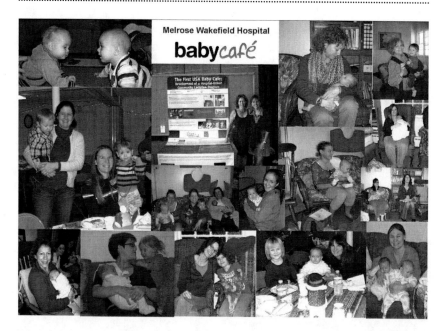

Figure 9.2. The first Baby Café in the United States at Melrose Wakefield Hospital.

HISTORY

In 2000 the first Baby Café breastfeeding drop-in support group was launched with UK Department of Health funding, specifically targeting vulnerable mothers. The project was delivered over the course of one year. We looked at where mums were already meeting locally, places that were comfortable, sociable, and easy to reach with a baby, toddler, and buggy. We decided to try to recreate that kind of atmosphere within a service that kept breastfeeding firmly as the focus. Tables were arranged as if in a café; clinical surroundings were disguised with purple throws, cushions, and attractive tablecloths. Drinks were served in china mugs. Posters and flyers were professionally designed and printed, giving a stylish look to this new service. We wanted the whole visual message to metaphorically shout that we valued what they were trying to do for their babies. A venue was carefully considered, as, although the service was open to all, we were determined that the harder-to-reach mothers would feel able to access the service. Mothers began to attend, and we tested our hypothesis, which was that mothers would continue to breastfeed if two essential elements were in place in one location. First, that any difficulties could be quickly identified and management strategies put in place immediately, and second, that other mothers who were going through similar events could help, support, and encourage each other.

We know that mothers learn more about breastfeeding by absorbing information from each other and their babies than can be found in any reference book. Breastfeeding is as much about the "art" and relationships as the physiological and biological aspects (Morbacher & Kendall-Tackett, 2005; Hoddinott, Kroll, Raja, & Lee, 2010). The aspiration at a Baby Café was to construct an environment for mothers where they could learn about breastfeeding by tuning in to their natural instincts, alongside access to skilled, one-to-one help when clinical challenges arose. The care that is given focuses on enabling a mother to learn about breastfeeding her own baby, rather than inundating her with a list of instructions (Figures 9.3, 9.4).

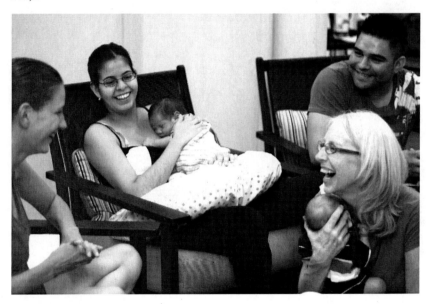

Figure 9.3. Baby Café in El Paso, Texas.

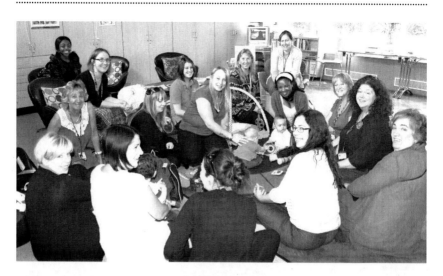

Figure 9.4. Potters Bar Baby Café, United Kingdom.

Evaluation of the project demonstrated that a wide reach of mothers accessed the service and found it helpful in supporting them to establish breastfeeding and continue to breastfeed (Pardoe & Williams, 2000). The project was included as a case study in the National Health Service Good Practice and Innovation in Breastfeeding document (Dykes, 2003; Department of Health, 2004). As a result of the project, the local health authority re-commissioned the service, and during the second year, additional funding was sought to train breastfeeding peer supporters by recruiting mothers who had used the service. The advantages of this were that mothers had already experienced the benefits of the Baby Café and that supervision and reflective practice were easier to manage.

Because of this, interest grew from other regions in the UK that wanted advice on how to set up their own Baby Cafés, so we developed guidelines and protocols to help them. After we established our website, inquiries came from further afield, and our first overseas Baby Café was set up in New Zealand. During that first year, some key issues and ways of working were identified, which became the foundation for the model of care that was tested, and then replicated around the country over the next 10 years. This was based on and continues to be informed by current research, evidence-based practice, and a culture of breastfeeding and client views (Dykes & Griffiths, 1998; Hoddinott & Roisin, 1999; Parker & Williams, 2000; Dykes, 2003; Dyson et al., 2006; Hoddinott, Britten, & Pill, 2010).

The Baby Café health professional-led model is based on the rationale that health professionals are effective at reaching mothers from every socio-economic, ethnic, and educational group as part of delivering maternity and post-natal care, and so they are well placed to provide an inclusive service. To date Baby Café has supported over 50,000 breastfeeding mothers throughout the UK (BCCT Annual Reports, 2012).

Staff and volunteers working in Baby Cafés have the opportunity to share local good practice, so service delivery across Baby Café drop-ins continues to be developed and improved. Examples of these developments include working in rural areas, producing translated materials, encouraging antenatal attendance, and managing health and safety issues to ensure that young mothers want to access the drop-in. The right mix of staff within a Baby Café is crucial to the success and sustainability of service delivery, and although perhaps not a qualification usually listed, we believe that those with a heart for breastfeeding mothers run thriving Baby Cafés. Many of our breastfeeding peer supporters are mothers who accessed the service for social contact or help in overcoming difficulties, and then had a strong desire to give something back to the service, as well as offering their support to the new mums coming in.

> MOTHER'S QUOTE: "It was a fantastic support to me—the professional and peer advice, as well as the sociable atmosphere."

Typically, a Baby Café is facilitated by a health professional. In the UK this is often a midwife or health visitor with extra professional development in breastfeeding. International Board Certified Lactation Consultants (IBCLC) also facilitate in Baby Cafés in both the UK and other countries. So alongside the informal and relaxed atmosphere is the professional aspect of a fully funded drop-in center with paid staff and the associated commitment this engenders.

As consumers we were aware that other organizations "brand" their products or services, so the Baby Café, with its distinctive branding, is becoming synonymous with breastfeeding, excellence, quality, and style, all within a relaxed and informal atmosphere. The Baby Café name is a registered trademark in the UK, USA, and France to ensure that the concepts and ethos of a friendly, relaxed atmosphere, with expert help and support always on hand, remain with the name. Brand recognition often helps practitioners secure funding and it attracts mothers.

NEW OPPORTUNITIES AND THE FUTURE

At the beginning of 2011, Baby Café merged with the NCT Group, a large UK-based parenting charity, to pool personnel, expertise, and contacts under another successful brand in order to take community-based breastfeeding support to many more mothers. In May 2011 we launched a new service called Baby Café Local with the NCT. Baby Café Local aims to extend the model and test different approaches to delivering the service, while still embodying the key concepts and ethos of Baby Café. Using the same rigorous application process developed for Baby Cafés, the aim is to look at a more flexible model in terms of staffing, open hours, and blocks of service delivery to see if it is possible to extend the model and still have the excellent breastfeeding rates and levels of satisfaction of this service. Applications to set up a Baby Café Local are invited from accredited breastfeeding practitioners from the NCT, La Leche League, the Association of Breastfeeding Mothers, and the Breastfeeding Network, as well as health workers who can demonstrate a high level of professional development in breastfeeding.

Part of the application process includes an induction day that outlines the benefits of operating under the brand and how the charity can help each Baby Café Local deliver the service. The opportunity is open to practitioners wanting to set up a new initiative and to those with existing breastfeeding services and drop-in groups.

There is already a growing number of Baby Café Locals, mainly in children's centers that are committed to joint partnership work and are well supported by staff who have the local knowledge and skills to work with more vulnerable families. (A children's center provides a single place for five key services: early education, childcare, health, family support, and help into work. They serve children and their families from conception until the children start primary education.)

We expect that Baby Café Local staff will be comfortable to work alongside health professionals and support cross referral systems that enable mothers and babies to be referred for community-based support routinely, and enable those needing additional support or care to be referred on to relevant services. In one area a cluster of four Baby Café Locals are all facilitated by NCT breastfeeding counselors supported by children's center staff, with a project manager in place to oversee the service and liaise with the charity. A children's center manager who attended a Baby Café Local induction day says,

> It's such a relief to know that we're in good hands by investing in a tried and tested service that has been delivering outcomes throughout the country for over 10 years. Baby Café Local will build on our existing services and relationships with local health

professionals, give value for money, and reach women at the margins of society.

NCT practitioners who have set up a Baby Café Local feel enthusiastic about the new opportunities. Cathy Harvey, NCT breastfeeding counselor at Baby Café Local Colburn, Catterick Garrison, says, "It's a big learning curve and I'm so enjoying the experience of working with women from a background I've not come across before within NCT. It's great to be able to use all my NCT training, skills, and resources alongside what the peer supporters and children's center staff bring to the team."

Those of us working in this area know how generous mothers can be and how much they want to give back. Baby Café Locals are ideally placed as a resource for recruiting volunteers, peer supporters, and new breastfeeding counselors who will all contribute to the cycle of support. Baby Café Local is a prime opportunity to extend the reach of breastfeeding support and a wide range of outcomes are measured as part of the on-going monitoring and evaluation that all drop-ins are supported to put in place. It is not always about numbers. Even one vulnerable mother who decides to give breastfeeding a go will be a powerful influence within a community whose prevailing culture is to use formula feeding, and this should be seen as a measure of success.

BARRIERS

Many Baby Cafés face the same challenges worldwide, that is, provision of ongoing funding. For services to become mainstream and be seen as an acceptable part of the provision of maternity and postnatal community care, they have to become evident as a standard part of the local healthcare scene, something that everyone finds easily available. Globally, many different healthcare systems are constantly challenged when it comes to allocating funds, and most are under pressure to deal with immediate healthcare issues rather than invest in long-term health benefits.

CONCLUSION

Much has been learned since 2000, and we find ourselves constantly evolving as more evidence presents itself to support the case for breastfeeding and as healthcare and commissioning services change (Renfrew et al., 2005; National Institute for Health and Clinical Excellence, 2006; Britten, McCormick, Renfrew, Wade, & King, 2007; Department of Health/ Department for Children, Schools, and Families, 2009; Department of Health, 2010; Marmot, 2010). As the organization grows, we are coming into contact with incredibly creative individuals whose professional artistry has helped to develop and evolve Baby Café from its first inception. At the center of all of this are the mothers. Their desire to do the best for their babies, to overcome difficulties, to give honest feedback about what helps, and perhaps more importantly what doesn't, provides us with the energy and enthusiasm to continue improving and developing services so that all mothers have access to the information and help they need to breastfeed.

Chapter Ten

International Organizations and the Mother-to-Mother Support Group

Maryanne Stone-Jimenez, MSc, IBCLC, LCCE
Judiann McNulty, MSc, DrPH

In 2001, Gaston Bozie, Regional Health Educator and Chairman of the Upper East Red Cross in Northern Ghana, said at the closing ceremony of the Mother Leaders Exchange meeting:

> I used to like getting large groups of women together and talking to them about health. I was skeptical of mother-to-mother support groups, but now I see their value. When you go back to your communities, don't worry about quantity. Worry about quality. It doesn't mean that health talks and health education will end. But when you're participating in mother-to-mother support groups, remember: no standing, no lectures, no knowing it all. These groups are for sharing information. And finally, remember to think Circle, Circle.

This meeting took place after a five-day training of local NGOs in northern Ghana on *Mother-to-Mother Support Group Methodology and Breastfeeding and Complementary Feeding Basics.*

Many NGOs and international organizations have implemented the targeted formation of community support groups facilitated by peer mothers instead of the mother-to-mother mentoring that takes place over an extended period of time in conventional support groups. They have sought to quicken the process by training peer mothers/facilitators in the content of breastfeeding and young child feeding (for the child under two years), support group methodology, and group dynamics. The power of the story, a cornerstone of conventional support groups, has become a new-found intervention, activity, and strategy in improving child feeding practices in developing countries.

Stories and fables have always provided a way to teach and pass on history, knowledge, norms, traditions, humor, and skills. When we share stories, we offer each other social and emotional support, empathy, respect, trust, and caring. Stories help us bridge the gap between knowledge, intuition, and feeling with the heart. There is power in storytelling. Support Groups are about stories. In the breastfeeding and young child feeding support group, pregnant women, mothers, grandmothers, and sisters come together to share their own stories about pregnancy and childbirth experiences, feeding their babies, and feeding their toddlers, and share in "watching their child grow." Out of shared stories grows the satisfaction of helping each other and learning that there is value in what "we are doing." Sharing stories in a support group gives women the determination and skills to exert control over their lives. The story enhances the perception of control. A support group helps to socially promote the "I can." Someone once said: "If you think you can or you can't, you're usually right." Support groups build the "I can," and lead to the empowering concept that "if she/they can, I can, too."

International organizations and Ministries of Health have adopted the support group methodology to promote exclusive breastfeeding in environments where cultural norms influence young women to introduce solid foods or other liquids too early or where "modernization" leads them to bottle feed. The support groups in these contexts are often linked with the Baby-Friendly Hospital Initiative as the 10th Step in certification; that is, assuring that mothers have access to support and guidance once they leave the hospital with their newborn.

Mercy Corps, an international NGO, recently started a program targeting the poorest districts of Jakarta, Indonesia. The Jakarta Provincial Health Department, with the Ministry of Social Welfare and Family Empowerment, is now expanding support groups throughout the city. The following story (Mercy Corps, 2009) illustrates the impact of support group participation on a young woman living in the crowded, unsanitary conditions of North Jakarta.

> When I had my first baby, I wanted so much to breastfeed him, but nobody supported my will because I was sick with a respiratory illness. The doctor and my relatives insisted that I should bottle-feed my baby. So, I bottle-fed my first baby from the day he was born, and he fell ill very frequently. He died due to severe diarrhea (Lena).

Lena (28 years) burst into tears when she shared her story in a Mother Support Group meeting in Tugu Utara Sub-district. Tugu Utara is the first sub-district in Jakarta Province that established a mother support group at the community level. With full support and participation of the sub-district authorities, local Health Centers, and community leaders, Mercy Corps started mother support groups in Tugu Utara sub-district by training 12 mothers in their 20s and 30s to become Breastfeeding Motivators. The mother support group is a safe, trusted, and friendly environment for young mothers like Lena to share personal experience, fears, doubts, tips, and information regarding child-care, with emphasis on breastfeeding.

Facilitated by trained Motivators, mother support group participants (i.e., pregnant and breastfeeding women) learn best practices from experiences shared among them, like the one Lena did.

> Learning from my experience with my first son, I insisted on breastfeeding my second baby despite my family's disapproval. I'm happy to see my daughter is growing up healthy and active. I want to help my friends in this group to successfully breastfeed their babies like I do.

Participation in mother support groups has motivated many young women in Tugu Utara sub-district to practice optimal breastfeeding. Moreover, many of these mothers have expressed interest in becoming Motivators, as they want more mothers in their neighborhoods to get the chance to learn what they have learned in mother support groups.

For women who have little education or opportunity to leave their homes, the mother support groups help build their self-esteem and their ability to interact with the larger world. The following are some examples of "I can" stories from women who participated in the La Leche League International Child Survival Project in Honduras where mothers from the peri-urban areas were trained as support group facilitators.

> The best experience in my life has been attending these meetings (support groups). For the first time in my life I feel like I am important.

> Before, when they asked for volunteers to read in my church, I wanted to, but I shook all over.... When I began to participate in the groups, I began to feel brave and now I always read. I don't feel afraid or embarrassed anymore.

Individual studies, including the evaluation of the Mercy Corps Jakarta project, show that support groups do not provide community-wide impact. However, direct participation within the support group has demonstrated behavior change. In the community-based mother-to-mother support group project with La Leche League Guatemala and in operational research conducted in the peri-urban areas of Guatemala City, it was shown that women who attended support groups were twice as likely to exclusively breastfeed their infants.

At present, capacity-building activities in many international and local non-government organizations incorporate a mother-to-mother support group component or intervention in their programming. This includes:

- A 5-day *Mother-to-Mother Support Group Methodology and Breastfeeding and Complementary Feeding Basics* curriculum (Academy for Educational Development LINKAGES, 2003).

- An instructional plan, training design, agenda, training materials.

- Field practice in facilitating support groups.

- A simple system of monitoring.

- Development of action plans.

- Assignment of responsibilities to continue supporting and forming community-based mother-to-mother support groups.

The curriculum and the mother-to-mother support groups address the pattern of breastfeeding, the adequate management of breastfeeding difficulties and techniques, and age-appropriate complementary feeding with local, available, feasible, seasonal, and affordable foods. Community-based mother-to-mother support groups addressing infant and young child feeding provide peer counseling within a supportive group setting and encourage mothers and caregivers to identify and solve their own infant and young child feeding difficulties. This non-formal education and experiential learning approach allows women to examine their values and attitudes, discover assumptions and patterns of behavior, ask questions, and re-learn new ways of thinking. Support groups empower women and caregivers to make better decisions and build self-confidence.

During the evaluation at the end of the Mother-to-Mother Support Group Training in Dadabb, the following questions and responses were given.

1. How has your idea of mother-to-mother support groups been changed or modified?

   ◊ "Facilitator should talk less."

◊   "Facilitator shares experience and gets/gives confidence to others."

◊   "Mother-to-mother support group can be a mix of pregnant and breastfeeding mothers."

◊   "Mother-to-mother support groups are not an educational talk, lecture, or class."

◊   "In a mother-to-mother support group, there is eye contact, sitting arrangement is in a circle with everyone at the same level."

2. What did you learn in the practice session of facilitating mother-to-mother support groups in the community?

◊   "It is difficult to change myths, but they can be overcome more in small groups."

◊   "When the facilitator shares her own experience, the group becomes open."

◊   "Confidence to train."

◊   "Very easy to manage a small group of six to eight, and hard to manage a larger group of 15."

◊   "Facilitator has to listen more."

3. Do you feel ready to facilitate Mother-to-Mother Support Groups in infant and young child feeding? Why?

◊   "We have captured the responsibilities of the facilitator."

◊   "We have received IYCF (infant and young child feeding) training and mother-to-mother support group training—we have knowledge and experience; we have seen how it is done."

To meet the needs of mothers, infants, and young children in an emergency setting, such as in Dadaab, access to basic infant and young child feeding and peer-to-peer support has been established by providing secure and supportive places (designated shelters, baby corners or mother-baby tents, child-friendly spaces) for mother/caregivers of infants and young children. This offers privacy for breastfeeding mothers (important for a displaced population or those in transit) and enables mother-to-mother support.

An observation form has been developed for use during on-going mentoring or supportive supervision. Simple pictorial forms have been designed to capture support group attendance of pregnant women, mothers who are breastfeeding, babies, other women, grandmothers and caregivers, and fathers. Figure 10.1 provides the Observation Checklist used for IYCF Support Groups and Figure 10.2 reproduces the IYCF Support Group Attendance pictorial form. Both materials are from the UNICEF

Community IYCF Counselling Package developed by UNICEF and URC. Figure 10.3 provides an example of a breastfeeding success story.

Figure 10.1. Observation Checklist for IYCF Support Groups

Figure 10. 1. Observation Checklist for IYCF Support Groups		
Community:	**Place:**	
Date: **Time:**	**Theme:**	
Name of IYCF Group Facilitator(s):	**Name of Supervisor:**	
--- ---	--- ---	
Did	✓	**Comments**
1. The Facilitator(s) introduce themselves to the group?		
2. The Facilitator(s) clearly explain the day's theme?*		
3. The Facilitator(s) ask questions that generate participation?		
4. The Facilitator(s) motivate the quiet women/men to participate?		
5. The Facilitator(s) apply skills for *Listening and Learning, Building Confidence and Giving Support*		
6. The Facilitator(s) adequately manage content?		
7. Mothers/fathers/caregivers share their own experiences?		
8. The Participants sit in a circle?		
9. The Facilitator(s) invite women/men to attend the next IYCF support group (place, date and theme)?		
10. The Facilitator(s) thank the women/men for attending the IYCF support group?		
11. The Facilitator(s) ask women to talk to a pregnant woman/man or breastfeeding mother before the next meeting, share what they have learned, and report back?		
12. Support Group attendance form checked?		
Number of women/men attending the IYCF support group:		
Supervisor/Mentor: indicate questions and resolved difficulties:		
Supervisor/Mentor: provide feedback to Facilitator(s):		

*The day's theme might change if there is a mother who has a feeding issue that she feels an urgent need to discuss.

Figure 10.2. IYCF Support Group Attendance Pictorial Form

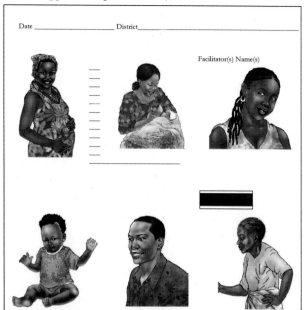

Figure 10.3. Example of Breastfeeding Success Story

(Printed in Mother Support Task Force: MSTF Volume 7, Number 2, May-August 2009)

Barni Ali Mohammed feels that receiving training in infant and young child feeding was very helpful to her. She had home deliveries of seven children, who were all given water with sugar until the third day when breastfeeding was initiated. The babies would fall sick often and were mostly admitted to the Supplementary Feeding Programme (SFP). In the training, she learnt about the importance of early initiation of breastfeeding, exclusive breastfeeding, and timely complementary feeding. When Abdiladif, her eighth child, was born, she observed these optimal IYCF practices and noticed a great difference in this child compared to her other children. She said, "When I was pregnant with Abdiladif, I also joined a mother-to-mother support group in my block from where I learnt a lot on appropriate infant and young child feeding practices. Abdiladif was delivered in the hospital and I breastfed him within 20 minutes after birth. No other foods or drinks were given to Abdi. I gave him only breastmilk for the first six months, and then introduced him to other foods after six months; he first refused to eat, but when a little breastmilk was added to the food, he ate it comfortably. I can say that he is different from the others, as he is very alert and he has never been sick or admitted to the hospital or any feeding programmes."

Barni Ali Mohammed has been able to reinforce these practices through the Mother-to-Mother support group where she is the group leader.

The formation of mother-to-mother support groups has become not only an intervention or activity within the international and local NGOs, but part of the global IYCF strategy that many countries have adopted for scaling up child health interventions and reaching the mother, father, caregiver, and family. The formation of mother-to-mother support groups in many countries is part of the national cascade of IYCF training as outlined in Figure 10.4 below. It is important that mother-to-mother support groups are part of the national training strategy and have national and international/local NGO "buy-in." The primary audience is the mother/father/caregiver/family and the cascade allows for two-way supportive supervision and mentoring at each level as depicted in the flowchart.

Figure 10.4. National Cascade of IYCF Training

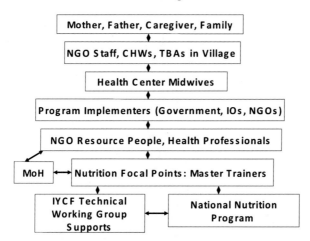

International and local NGOs and country IYCF strategies have succeeded in structuring and systematizing conventional mother-to-mother support groups into a replicable concept model describing steps of start-up and maintenance, support group activities, and desirable outcomes (Figure 10.5).

Figure 10.5. Concept Model for Mother-to-Mother Support Groups

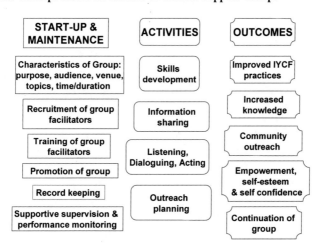

In the concept model structured above, there are continuing challenges at each of the three steps—particularly supportive supervision and performance monitoring, development and application of listening-dialoguing-acting skills, and group continuation. Organizations and country strategies are responding uniquely to these challenges, while focusing on the support group as a definite means of changing infant and young child feeding practices.

One of the major challenges is shifting the paradigm of health personnel and NGO staff who are not familiar with the peer support methodology. They often struggle to accept that there is no "teacher" nor "messages," but rather that the mothers can learn from each other. There is also the challenge of giving enough support to the facilitators to enable them to develop good facilitation skills, something that may take more time than is available in a time-limited project.

Implementation of support groups has not always met with success. In rural Nicaragua, the mothers simply lived too far apart to come to meetings. In a Malawi program where women met on the day they received donated food, they ceased participating as soon as the food distribution ended. In Azerbaijan, where women are generally well educated, the mothers rejected the idea of learning from each other and requested more formal lessons with discussion afterwards.

The international organizations are now looking at how to sustain the successful groups over time after project support has ended. One strategy is to link the facilitators with local health staff for on-going support, requiring the health staff to report to the health director on the continuation of the group. Another model in Peru has created a loose organization of the support group facilitators in one mountain region with the expectation that they will support each other to continue with the groups.

Part III: Moving Forward: Overcoming Barriers to Mother Support

Chapter Eleven

Beyond the 10th Step: The WABA Agenda to Broaden Mother Support Worldwide

Sarah Amin, MA
Rebecca Magalhães
Paulina Smith

BACKGROUND

As has been stated in earlier chapters, the 10th Step is critical to successful breastfeeding to ensure that a mother receives support for breastfeeding immediately after discharge from the hospital. However, continued postnatal support, including when the mother returns to work, is also very important, as is the period during pregnancy and birth.

Mother support in the context of the 10th step of the Baby-Friendly Hospital Initiative (BFHI) has traditionally been perceived as support provided in a mother support group (MSG) setting. The organizations that practiced the mother support group strategy at the time of the initiation of BFHI were mainly mothers helping mothers (mother-to-mother support). These support groups took place in the community and welcomed women into the group—before pregnancy, during pregnancy, after the birth, until the baby ceased breastfeeding, and even after. One way in which hospitals have complied with the 10th Step has been to set up support groups in the hospital or maternity facility setting, utilizing their own staff and thereby limiting the effectiveness of this Step. This approach has not been completely effective; whereas mother support groups go beyond the period the mother is in the hospital, and the need for support continues after she returns home.

It has long been known that a woman needs various kinds of support—from the health facility, the home, the workplace, and the community—to ensure that she is able to breastfeed successfully. The earlier chapters have talked extensively about support needed from the health system, which is important. International documents, such as the 1990 Innocenti Declaration and the 2003 *Global Strategy for Infant and Young Child Feeding* (GSIYCF), recognize the need for supporting mothers. However, no international document has put mother support in terms of a specific target to be achieved, nor has it been precisely defined. Given this, it is not surprising that when the global community, in the early 1990s and after, looked at why, despite a number of international policies and programs to support breastfeeding, it was observed that women still found it a challenge to practice and sustain exclusive breastfeeding for six months, and continue breastfeeding thereafter. (With BFHI, it was assumed that Step 10 or the mother support group is automatically there for the hospitals to tap in to, but this may not be the case. Thus mother support, especially mother support groups, needed to be systematically organized, trained, linked, funded, and supported.) In a continuing review of the state of breastfeeding through the years, the World Alliance for Breastfeeding Action (WABA) identified strategic areas of action that needed reinforcing, one of which has been mother support. From its inception, WABA set up the Mother Support Task Force as the vehicle through which this reinforcement could be provided.

HISTORY OF MOTHER SUPPORT WORK IN WABA

The First Decade: Strengthening Mother Support Groups, Mother-To-Mother Support and Beyond

In 1992 when the World Alliance for Breastfeeding Action was founded, the Mother Support Group Task Force was among the first task forces to be established. However, it was soon renamed as the Mother-to-Mother Support (MTMS) Task Force to give global significance and value to mother-to-mother support, which until then was undervalued internationally.

For the first decade, the WABA MTMS Task Force, led and coordinated by La Leche League International (LLLI) representatives, focused on interacting with and strengthening existing mother support groups (MSGs), while encouraging the development of new ones. The MTMS Task Force worked to link traditional MTMS groups with other breastfeeding groups practicing mother support to increase networking in the global breastfeeding movement. One example of such an action was the production of the Mother-to-Mother Support Activity Sheet #2, in English and Spanish (Figure 11.1). This was widely distributed by WABA and other organizations. Historically, from a network building perspective, mother support organizations and groups have generally been isolated, underfunded, and invisible in comparison to other kinds of breastfeeding organizations and have received minimal global recognition. Even La Leche League International, with community groups in over 50 countries, was not generally respected for its work with breastfeeding. This may be due to their localized nature, as well as their not having a focus on public advocacy. Therefore, the goal of the WABA Mother Support program in this first decade was to facilitate the development and visibility of mother support groups located in various places around the world, while facilitating a platform for these groups to connect, exchange experiences, and organize. In addition, the WABA mother support program pursued and reinforced a broader definition of mother support towards the end of the first decade, as greater networking of mother support organizations and other support groups occurred.

Figure 11.1. Online Resources

World Alliance for Breastfeeding Action (WABA): http://www.waba.org.my
Mother-to-Mother Support Activity Sheet #2 (English and Spanish): http://www.waba.org.my/resources/activitysheet/acsh2.htm
The Men's Initiative, which includes the Global Initiative for Father Support (GIFA): http://www.waba.org.my/whatwedo/mensinitiative/index.htm
Global Initiative for Mother Support, GIMS+5 Statement: http://www.waba.org.my/whatwedo/gims/gims+5.htm weblink)
GIMS e-map: http://www.waba.org.my/whatwedo/gims/emap.htm
Breastfeeding Gateway: http://breastfeedinggateway.org

In line with this second aim, the task force underwent another change in identity towards the latter part of the decade and renamed itself as the Mother Support Task Force. WABA recognized that while mother-to-mother support is a significant way through which women receive and give support on breastfeeding, women benefit from many different kinds of support. These include family, workplace, community, legal, and governmental, all of which create an enabling environment. A comment from WABA's consultations with a network participant summarizes this very well:

> Moral and social support is needed from many persons in different places. Women need the support of professional health providers, employers, friends, family, and the community. Conditions need to be created during pregnancy, birth, and lactation so that women can safely carry healthy babies to term and give birth in the company of those they select to share this experience. Employed women should receive support for

practicing exclusive breastfeeding for the first six months, and continued breastfeeding after the introduction of complementary foods (WABA, 2001).

Support to breastfeed comes from practically anywhere or anyone—men, friends, family, doulas, colleagues, employers, even the postman! Of course, each actor provides support specific to his or her capacity, skill, or knowledge level, but cumulatively it has a positive, multipronged effect for the woman. WABA's 1996 World Breastfeeding Week (WBW) theme on "Breastfeeding: A Community Responsibility" reflected this broad approach to supporting a mother (Figure 11.2).

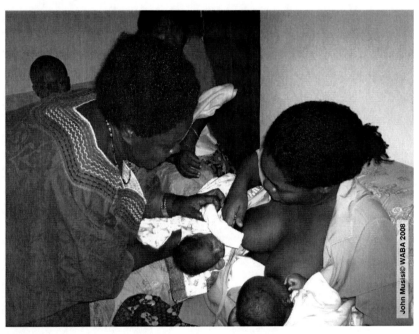

Figure 11.2. One-on-one support from within the family helps a new mother get off to a good start. (Photo by John Musisi, © WABA 2008.)

The Second Decade: Expanding The Scope To A Woman's Reproductive Continuum

Mother support organizations (such as La Leche League International, the Nursing Mothers Association of Australia, now known as the Australian Breastfeeding Association, and Ammehjelpen and Amningshjälpen in Norway and Sweden) have always practiced breastfeeding support as a continuous process (from pregnancy, birth, the postpartum period, and infant and toddler breastfeeding). On the other hand, public health initiatives generally treat breastfeeding as starting at birth. Furthermore, as the name implies, the BFHI focuses on the baby and does not sufficiently address the needs of women. Evidence has increased of the link between reduced intervention in birthing practices and better breastfeeding outcomes. These positive outcomes happen when women are supported during the birth process, have natural births, and have doulas or women supporting them during their birth and afterwards to help care for them and to support breastfeeding. By the turn of the century, WABA recognized the global need to take into account the woman's reproductive continuum from pregnancy, birth, and to the postpartum period, including breastfeeding, and to put the strength of the WABA global network behind a push to broaden the global discourse on mother support. Thus the first decade of the MSTF focused on expanding the notion of mother support beyond mother-to-mother support to other kinds of support, while strengthening the global network for mother support groups. The second decade spearheaded the concept of mother support throughout the reproductive continuum from pre-pregnancy, pregnancy, and birth to breastfeeding.

GLOBAL INITIATIVE FOR MOTHER SUPPORT (GIMS)

This effort was accomplished through *The Global Initiative for Mother Support (GIMS) for Breastfeeding*, born in 2000, when two representatives from the USAID funded project "LINKAGES" travelled to Malaysia to meet with WABA staff and members of a local mother support organization on a proposal for a mother support conference. A preliminary outline for a GIMS statement was composed as a meeting outcome and further developed through an innovative online discussion with about 63 participants. This statement was finalized and became the topic of a one-day meeting at the 2001 LLLI International Conference. By 2002, with GIMS already a reality, two regional conferences launched it. The first GIMS conference was held in Malaysia for the Asia Pacific region, with the theme of supporting working women, in order to link the two aspects of supporting mothers and working women. This was followed by a similar event in Peru for the Latin American region. Finally, GIMS had a significant presence at the WABA Global Forum II in Arusha, Tanzania, where it was launched to the wider global breastfeeding network and UN representatives present.

An initial and innovative on-line discussion on GIMS was critical to the process of exploring the depth and expansiveness of mother support as a concept and practice, and at arriving at a common understanding on the

GIMS as a global initiative.[5] The discussion helped to define mother support, come up with a name for the Initiative, and define its scope, purpose, goals, and focus. A sampling of the participants' responses/inputs is compiled here in quotes to give the reader a sense of the evolution and thinking around mother support and the GIMS.

When the participants were asked what came to their minds with the phrase "support for women," these were the main responses:

> Help, listening, practical information, practical help, empowerment, culturally appropriate, nutritional support, moral support, empathy, sharing, respect, money, resources, kindness, gentleness, paid maternity leave of six months, understanding, counseling, access to skilled breastfeeding management.

To receive the level of help required, mothers and babies need much, much more than just "support." Mothers and babies need face-to-face, individualized hands-on assistance, information, teaching, and techniques by skilled practitioners specifically trained in breastfeeding and lactation management techniques, tailor-made to the unique and particular difficulty or situation.

Mother support has come to mean information, encouragement, affirmation, very valuable contact with other mothers, and a sort of group visual aid, so that less experienced mothers can observe more experienced mothers in the tried and tested technique of using one mother to educate another on how normal, natural breastfeeding takes place and evolves from one stage of babyhood to the next. It may also mean legislation and practices which allow breastfeeding mothers to maintain breastfeeding, such as protection for working mothers (e.g., maternity leave, breastfeeding/pumping breaks while at work) or protection for breastfeeding in public places.

In the context of "pregnancy, birth, and lactation," mother support would mean creating conditions in which women can safely carry (healthy) babies to term, give birth in the company of those people they select to share this experience, and be together with their babies enough to ensure that six months exclusive breastfeeding and on-going breastfeeding after the introduction of complementary foods is possible. It also means:

---

5   This online discussion, or e-dialogue, took place among a number of individuals round the world in 2001. The e-dialogue was a series of unpublished, personal communications, as was a later e-dialogue.

- Nutritional support during pregnancy and lactation where and when household food insecurity occurs.

- Moral support from friends and family and the community achieved through positive and supportive social norms.

- Ensuring appropriate care for women from those involved with her before and after her baby's birth—full communication, ensuring accurate and relevant information is provided, and respectful treatment and support given for the choices she makes.

From health services and the community, mother support would mean:

- Ensuring that there is both the necessary range of professional health services for mothers, infants, and young children and adequate peer support in the community, so mothers have the tools they need to nourish their children's bodies and nurture their spirits.

- Healthcare service support (indicating that this includes not just improving healthcare workers' knowledge and skills in breastfeeding and childbirth management, but striving to change the inhumane "bedside manner" that seems to be the norm by all but midwives in most countries).

For the working mother:

- Support for working women to be with the newborn for at least six months through paid leave with public funds, not the employer.

- Support for working women to continue breastfeeding through paid breastfeeding breaks and hygienic facilities for feeding or expressing/ pumping milk up to one year after birth, paid through public funds.

From other entities/organizations, it means:

- Concrete government support and implementation of initiatives which would provide the optimal environment for breastfeeding—WHO Code, BFHI, relevant ILO conventions, legislation to protect the rights of women who are breastfeeding.

In terms of dissemination of information, mother support implies:

- Providing partners, support networks and the general community with information and education about the support needed by mothers and encouraging them to become active participants in this process.

- Ensuring appropriate extent and quality of breastfeeding education.

In "special circumstances," mother support is needed for ill or disabled mothers and for those mothers with premature infants or with infants and children who are ill or disabled.

More generally, mother support also implies:

- Working to eliminate barriers to breastfeeding, whether they be financial, environmental, or attitudinal.

- Valuing lactation.

- Actively promoting and funding of mother-to-mother support groups where they exist.

- Utilizing GIMS human rights language in presenting these needs for support.

The Initiative is not about mother-to-mother support. It is about supporting mothers (mother support). This is a very important distinction. This is what is going to give this Initiative the creativity on the many different ways a mother can/needs to be/should be supported. It is about "the many faces of mother support" (Figure 11.3).

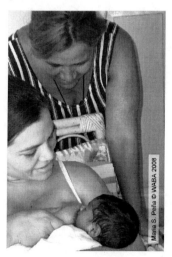

Figure 11.3. Mother support includes the encouragement of other women. (Photo by Maria S. Peña. © WABA 2008.)

One of the main goals of this Initiative is that it be flexible, adaptable, and aimed at satisfying the diversity of mothers' needs. The parameters will be broad (for this very same reason).

GIMS as an initiative recognizes the diversity of support needs. GIMS endorsers will/can choose what means of support they can best enhance or provide. Those engaging in GIMS actions may select from a list of approaches and ideas. Some groups may have the agenda of strengthening community support systems, while others will focus on mother-to-mother support. Still others may concentrate on the health or other sectors of the community.

The discussion also touched on the question of whether the focus of the GIMS should be on the reproductive cycle or on the fuller range, including the woman-girl child. Several participants were of the view that the GIMS seemed most reasonable if applied to the reproductive years, using the goals or preamble to recognize the importance of remembering the girl child. That is, not expanding the scope too much. Other participants felt strongly that WABA supports not only lactating women, but also the woman-girl, woman-adolescent, woman-woman, woman-mother, woman-grandmother, and woman-elderly. In other words, breastfeeding support is throughout the woman's life. It was felt by many that the span could be stretched from the time a girl-child reaches puberty, when her body is capable of pregnancy, until the woman reaches and passes through menopause.

On the FOCUS of support, comments included:

- Breadth is a prerequisite if GIMS is to include the creation of a social climate supportive of breastfeeding. Social norms will never be breastfeeding friendly unless someone works on it.

- From the inception of the GIMS, it was hoped that the Initiative would help the breastfeeding movement link more broadly with natural childbirth and parenting groups, as well as women's health organizations that focus on women's reproductive health.

- GIMS could include a category that focuses specifically on education. Here we could include the education and outreach needed to reach the girl-child all the way through to the older woman. This part of the Initiative could include volunteers who could work within a community to present breastfeeding and reproductive issues that relate to the success and promotion of breastfeeding as the norm. They would use whatever tools would be most effective in teaching within that particular community. Dolls for little children, posters, artwork, printed materials, etc. were all issues that have been brought up in the discussion so far. Several people have expressed the wish that these things were important tools they would like to see incorporated.

Finally, when the GIMS Statement was adopted, it defined the GIMS for Breastfeeding as follows:

> A global initiative that focuses on women's needs and rights to adequate and accurate information, support, and healthcare services before, during, and after childbirth. The initiative takes a holistic view of women's reproductive cycle and promotes various measures to help mothers and their infants experience optimal breastfeeding (WABA, 2002a).

It also defined "mother support" as:

> Any support provided to mothers for the purpose of improving breastfeeding practices for both mother and baby. The support needed varies from woman to woman, but generally includes encouragement, accurate and timely information, humane care during childbirth, advice, reassurance, affirmation, hands-on assistance, and practical tips (WABA, 2002a).

Its Vision is that:

> Every woman, irrespective of her circumstance of residence, will have lay, professional, and social support for breastfeeding and will receive the necessary information, education, and encouragement enabling her to have the breastfeeding experience she and her child want (WABA, 2002a).

The Statement declared among other pertinent positions, the following positions reflective of the expanded discourse on mother support:

- Mother support should be viewed and valued as an important contributor to optimal infant feeding practices *throughout the reproductive cycle*, with special attention on *humanizing pregnancy and childbirth care.*

- Mother support should be *defined broadly as any support* provided to mothers for the purpose of improving breastfeeding practices for both mother and baby. Mothers should receive support *throughout their entire reproductive cycle* (pregnancy, birthing, and post-natal; WABA, 2002a).

It is also critical to note that the GIMS is based on an approach that respects human rights and women's reproductive rights. This approach calls for *men's participation* and community involvement. In fact, the male participants at the WABA Global Forum II were inspired by the GIMS and set up a **Global Initiative for Father Support (GIFS)** (WABA, 2002b, p.

3). Thus the GIFS was launched at the same event with much excitement. The fathers who attended the Forum wanted to position themselves in the movement as a critical group for supporting mothers, as well as to support each other (men themselves) in implementing their role as fathers. Reclaiming fatherhood and the right to paternity were complementary issues. Sustaining the GIFS, however, has been a challenge for WABA for lack of a coordinated effort and committed on-going leadership. More recently, the GIFS has been couched under the broader action of the Men's Initiative (Figure 11.1).

IMPLEMENTING THE GIMS: MS e-NEWSLETTER, SEED GRANT PROJECT, AND OTHERS

Following the launch of the GIMS, the WABA Mother Support Task Force (MSTF) embarked on innovative efforts and activities to promote the GIMS as a new concept and initiative. This included the founding in 2003 of an electronic newsletter, titled the *MSTF e-Newsletter*. The main purpose of the e-newsletter is to keep GIMS endorsers in contact with each other. An additional purpose is to stimulate the ongoing involvement of new people and groups to practice and engage in mother support in a broad way, thereby linking them to the WABA network.

Since its founding, the *e-Newsletter* has been issued continually in three languages (English, Spanish, and French), with a fourth language (Portuguese), added in 2005, increasing WABA's outreach to populations that are not fluent in English. This publication provides an opportunity for people not only to learn from others about mother support, but to also share their experiences and knowledge on the subject for the benefit of others. As the years went by and in response to expressed needs, new sections and topics were added. Currently, the *e-Newsletter* contains the following: Mother Support Task Force Comments and Information, Mother Support from Different Sources, Breastfeeding Mothers Relate Their Experiences, Father Support, News from the Breastfeeding World, Breastfeeding Resources, Children and Breastfeeding, Grandmothers and Grandfathers Support Breastfeeding, Breastfeeding: HIV and AIDS, and Newsletter Information (Websites, Past and Future Events, Readers Share). The newsletter also honors special breastfeeding advocates who have promoted, protected, and supported breastfeeding in all parts of the world.

The newsletter soon became a virtual forum, producing a rich exchange of experiences and ideas from diverse stakeholders involved in mother support. To date, with direct and indirect subscribers, *the e-Newsletter* has an estimated global reach of 14,000 readers, and involves 50 or more contributors from different countries in each issue. Direct subscribers share the newsletter with their respective networks, resulting in this broader reach. In addition, the newsletter in all languages is posted on the Mother Support Task Force section of the WABA website, where more than 1,000 persons download each issue directly. The first issue in 2011 was translated for the first time into Arabic, and there is interest in a Chinese translation.

The *MSTF e-Newsletter* is one of the most successful outreach avenues thus far in the history of mother support worldwide, and continues to exist and to be in demand, despite diminished funding. The voluntary nature of mother support, in general, has kept this newsletter going so strongly over the past nine years. Hopefully, it will continue to be the engine for the outreach, even if no new funds are found. As has been said, one of the many benefits of the newsletter is the way in which persons, far-flung around the world, can learn about an activity, program, or effort that they may not have heard of. They can now connect to those who coordinate that particular activity, program, or effort. The networking potential provided by the newsletter makes it a valuable WABA asset.

In order to stimulate more specific father and community support measures worldwide, WABA started a small seed grant project that operated from 2003-2006, with each grant providing USD $500-$2000 to the grantee. Although over a hundred applications were received in each grant round, WABA could only allocate about eight to 10 grants in each round. The application process was overwhelming, not just in sheer volume, but also because the need expressed was great, and it would often be difficult to refuse those that didn't make the top eight or 10. What the grant process showed, in addition to the need, was the diverse creativity among communities in the different countries in offering support to breastfeeding mothers. Reports of several of the seed grants projects showed correlation between the support initiatives provided and increased breastfeeding practiced in the community.

The projects that targeted fathers, namely in Mozambique, Pakistan, Nepal, India, Sri Lanka, and Indonesia, had the primary goal of training men in communities to set up father support groups. The projects in Mozambique and India both targeted youth to start father support groups. The Indonesia project aimed to start father support groups in Bali among families suffering hardship because of economic decline after the terrorist bombings in 2002. Strategies of these three projects included a slogan/poster contest and exhibition, training of young male HIV counselors about exclusive breastfeeding and supporting mothers, designing and producing pamphlets and T-shirts, and sensitization for community members through debates, meetings, and workshops. The project in Nepal targeted workers, employers, and trade unionists in an industrial district. The Paraguay grant followed a different strategy, as these grantees set out to include information on father support in the GIMS newsletter and to do outreach about father support groups in Paraguay.

The Sudanese Breastfeeding Association (SABA) used the grant to develop three mother support groups which served to increase voluntary efforts to support exclusive breastfeeding in the community. Kindergartens were enlisted and upgraded with educational aids and materials to provide this support for the mother support groups. This project had value-added effects in seven villages, and the message extended to a wider locality. In Pakistan, the project established a network of large groups of women in the districts of Mansehra and Abbottabad to support optimal breastfeeding and young child feeding by sensitizing senior students of grades 13 and 14 and teachers of five higher educational institutions for women. It reached a primary audience of some 1800 senior female students and 89 female teachers. Every single student and teacher further communicated specifically taught messages to five close friends, neighbors, family members, and relatives, resulting in an outreach to almost 10,000 women (WABA, 2006). While the above two examples focused on schools in different ways, as channels for strengthening and furthering mother support, the other seed grant projects targeted an array of different agents of support. These included community leaders, the business community, women's groups, religious leaders, fathers, and even the postmen (mail carriers) in Brazil. All of them to some extent indicated increased interest, understanding, and uptake of better infant feeding practices. What would have been useful is on-going financial and related support for some of these projects, including monitoring of breastfeeding practices and rates in the defined communities for a certain period of time. Thus their outcomes would have been clearer.

RENEWING GLOBAL COMMITMENT ON MOTHER SUPPORT

GIMS +5, the e-Dialogue, and a Mother Support Summit

Five years after the official launching of the GIMS at the WABA Global Forum II, WABA recognized the need to renew global commitment and revive global action around mother support. It was also important to remind people that the GIMS was focused on the broad notion of diverse and multipronged support, as such a notion was not yet adequately internalized by a large global audience. LLLI was also interested in featuring the topic of mother support at its 50th Anniversary of the founding of LLLI. So, together, LLLI and WABA organized and implemented *The State of the Art of Mother Support Summit* in 2007, as a two-day meeting prior to the beginning of the LLLI 50th Anniversary Conference in Chicago, Illinois, USA.

What was important to the ultimate success of the Mother Support Summit was not just the program and the outcomes, but that an e-dialogue took place in the months before the event among potential conference participants and others who wanted to participate, but could not attend. The e-dialogue was implemented in order for the Summit to begin with much of the work and preparation accomplished, thereby increasing the possibility of a successful summit outcome. The dialogue covered a range of issues based on the following four key questions:

Question 1: In your experience or in your work, what element or component has been the most effective and positive influence on supporting the breastfeeding mother?

Question 2: In your opinion, what are the obstacles that hinder or impede a positive breastfeeding experience?

Question 3: In what way could we collaborate in order to get international recognition for the need for mother support?

Question 4: What do you think is the single most effective action worldwide for improving/ increasing mother support? (WABA-LLLI, 2007)

Each question was discussed for a period of two weeks, with a summary at the end of the two weeks for that particular question.

On QUESTION 1, regarding the most effective and positive influence on supporting the breastfeeding mother, the most pertinent response was *direct and immediate support*, even while many felt that the larger social environment, such as being in a breastfeeding culture or having experienced a breastfeeding tradition in the family were important factors. Examples of direct support given were "in mother support groups in a hospital setting, mother-to-mother support groups, other formal support groups, through peer counselors, midwives, a phone call, in person encouragement, a human touch, a helping hand, a caring and loving breastfeeding friendly environment." But such direct support needs an enabling political environment, and this needed to be formalized and propagated through national policy. To summarize what the group wants to see is "a global strategy that enables the breastfeeding mother to be supported at home, in health institutions, in the community, and in the workplace as a result of education, training, as well as national and local norms."

On QUESTION 2, the obstacles that impede a positive breastfeeding experience, five key elements were identified:

1. Aggressive marketing strategies by baby food and formula manufacturers.

2. Hospital practices that do not facilitate the mother getting off to a good breastfeeding relationship.

3. The doctor/physician who is unethical or uninformed.

4. The lack of accurate information available for the mother, as well as the lack of support.

5. Realities for the working mothers.

The first three elements are interrelated, with the baby food industry being a key factor influencing unsupportive healthcare practices and health professionals' ethical standards by inducing them with gifts and free samples. The result is confusing messages to mothers. Doctors are held in high regard and seen as a legitimate source of information, even when they are wrong; and it is even worse when they openly and unnecessarily prescribe infant formula. These three factors then lead to the fourth: Mothers do not receive accurate and adequate information and support from healthcare staff and have misconceptions about breastfeeding, ultimately practicing mixed feeding (breastmilk and formula). The lack of supportive conditions at work and lack of paid maternity leave add to these pressures, making it difficult for a woman to practice exclusive breastfeeding.

Getting international recognition for mother support as a practice has been a priority for WABA and the Mother Support Task Force. Hence QUESTION 3 sought collective ideas from the network to see how WABA could work towards this goal. The responses centered on *creating partnerships and advocacy* with a variety of international stakeholders. These included international agencies, such as WHO, ILO, the World Bank, UNICEF, governments, as well as targeting youth on a global level as future advocates, and *lobbying for funds*. The last item mentioned also included training key people to be alert to opportunities for funding sources. The advocacy aspect would involve convincing governments that support groups are necessary in every village and community and of the need to create an enabling environment for this. This would involve a range of actions. These include strengthening existing IYCF regulations and laws to aid these goals, effective workplace reforms, education of community populations on mother support, developing trainers and leaders in mother support (for example, through international accreditation programs for mother support group leaders), and other actions.

Information dissemination was yet another thrust proposed. Ideas included:

> Using media outlets, a campaign to have Surgeon Generals/ Ministers of Health put warnings on formula containers, campaign for the acceptance and support for mother support groups, ongoing positive stories, stories that humanize mother support groups in the public mind, and encouraging women who breastfeed to speak up—make them spokespeople for mother support.

Last but not least, on the single most effective action worldwide for improving/ increasing mother support, a two-pronged response was solicited to **QUESTION 4.** The first and all encompassing response was for mother support groups to be available to every mother, while the second was for the Baby-Friendly Hospital Initiative (BFHI) to improve and increase mother support worldwide. On the first aspect, again suggestions were made to "convince governments to create this force in every community, village, and town." This would require training and supporting the mother support leaders/peer counselors/health workers to facilitate the support groups, providing them with communication and negotiation skills, linking them with community-based organizations and health facilities, etc. The BFHI, as the second aspect, was seen as potentially having a positive influence that is far reaching on supporting mothers beyond the hospital environment, and thus furthering the first aspect. Quoting a participant, "The influence of BFHI on community practitioners and the community *per se* has set the platform.... The 10 Steps have an influence over the wider community. It is a vessel for raising the profile of breastfeeding in the community." Other related responses included the request for the implementation of mother support groups as a pre-requisite to any BFHI certification, including that maternity facilities make mothers aware of support available when they return home.

These four questions and the respective responses were brought to the Mother Support Summit for further discussion by the participants, who further dialogued on the above in five groups (WABA-LLLI, 2007). Perhaps the most significant addition to the dialogue was to Question 4, which ultimately became the main response for the single most effective action worldwide at that time. This was for the proposed theme for World Breastfeeding Week 2008 to be Mother Support to increase global advocacy and action on the topic.

Another important development at the Summit was to revisit and revise the GIMS Statement to update it and expand its endorsement. Here, the

GIMS+5 Statement was issued and received new endorsements (WABA, 2007b). The text used the original GIMS Statement as a starting point, with modifications and new elements or emphasis where needed.

The *vision* remained almost the same, with the additional recognition of women of ALL ages, ethnicity, religion, economic, social, and professional/ educational status. Meanwhile, the definition of mother support is elaborated below, mainly to emphasize the role of evidence-based health policies and research, as well as the multifaceted actors in mother support:

> Mother support is any support provided to mothers for the purpose of improving breastfeeding practices for both mother and infant and young child. *Women need the support of evidence-based public health policies, health providers, employers, friends, family, the community, and particularly that of other women and mothers.* The support needed varies from woman to woman, but generally includes accurate and timely information to help her build confidence; *sound recommendations based on up-to-date research; compassionate care* before, during, and after childbirth; *empathy and active listening;* hands-on assistance; and practical guidance.

The *Goals* of the GIMS+5 were also further developed and refined as follows:

- *To promote* a global understanding of mother support that values, gives credibility to, and actively strengthens all forms of mother support including community-based breastfeeding mother support programs and networks.

- *To broaden* the support for mothers to include: support before and during pregnancy, at birth, and during the breastfeeding period.

- *To link and collaborate* with other issue movements, such as those working on natural, compassionate childbirth and health practices, family support, midwifery, women's health and rights, youth, HIV and AIDS support groups, etc. in order to facilitate a holistic view of mother support which is respectful of the integrity of women's rights and the optimal health and survival of infants and young children.

- *To work* with interested organizations to develop guidelines, tools, and training for transforming birthing and healthcare practices that specifically affect breastfeeding and women's rights into compassionate and gender sensitive birthing and healthcare practices.

- *To support Step 10* of the Baby-Friendly Hospital Initiative (BFHI) by broadening the understanding of <u>breastfeeding support</u> and support groups, <u>being open to innovative ways to support the mother after birth.</u>

- *To initiate, act on, and support* changes in <u>public policies, cultural attitudes</u>, employment, health facilities, marketplace and <u>social policies and practices</u> so that women experience <u>optimal conditions to decide on their maternity</u>, pregnancy, birthing, and breastfeeding practices.

The texts underlined indicate the additions or new emphasis. It is clear that emphasis is given in the GIMS+5 Statement to further expanding the types of support women need, especially in view of the HIV pandemic where clearer policy guidance was needed based on public health rationale (Figure 11.4). A new emphasis in the Statement is also given to recognize the importance of public and social policy and practices and cultural attitudes in shaping a breastfeeding culture and to value increased attention to women's rights and the need to bring about conditions to support a woman's right to decide on matters concerning maternity, etc. (WABA, 2007c). It also makes special mention of youth as an important support group to be fostered, the result of the Global Summit's special program session that focused on youth and men as active agents in mother support.

Figure 11.4. GIMS +5 Statement on HIV and Infant Feeding

HIV and infant feeding policies were initially based on a public health rationale: HIV-infected mothers in industrialized countries were advised to formula-feed, whereas HIV infected mothers in developing countries were advised to continue breastfeeding. Then, from 1997 to 2006, recommendations for developing countries focused on private rights. Currently, due to research results demonstrating high malnutrition and mortality for formula-fed babies in developing countries, the 2006 revised HIV and infant feeding recommendations re-endorse a public health rationale in all settings, as follows:

- The most appropriate infant feeding option should continue to depend on a mother's individual circumstances, including her health status and the local situation, but should take greater consideration of available health services.

- Governments and other stakeholders should re-vitalize breastfeeding protection, promotion, and support in the general population and should also actively support HIV-infected mothers.

HIV-exposed infants should receive exclusive breastfeeding for the first 6 months of life and continued breastfeeding with additional complementary foods after 6 months unless replacement feeding is acceptable, feasible, affordable, sustainable, and safe.

While the 2002 GIMS Statement already called for promoting Step 10 of the BFHI, emphasis is given in GIMS+5 to broadening the understanding of *breastfeeding support* from the health facility perspective and promoting the concept of mother-friendly care practices related to compassionate birth and care of the mother, which should be women-centered. The BFHI with its focus on the baby, conceptually and practically, often leads health facilities to ignore the woman in the symbiotic act of breastfeeding. In the context of the GIMS, the BFHI would need to be more "mother-friendly." Pregnant women and those who have just given birth are often in a precarious situation due to fragmented services and lack of supportive policies, procedures, and practices in health facilities. A hospital which is also mother-friendly would require ensuring that antenatal, labor, delivery, and postnatal care for the mother supports women's health and well-being, recognizing that such care also supports optimal breastfeeding.

From a women-centered approach, even if a woman is breastfeeding, she should be doing so because she has the ability to decide on it and is getting the needed support on the various fronts, not because she is "forced" to do so or is without choice. The GIMS+5 Statement makes this very clear:

> It emphasizes gender-sensitive policies and support services, women's right to appropriate sexual and prenatal education and care, and women-centered birthing practices, all of which should give an appropriate and adequate measure of control to women over their bodies, health, and lives (WABA, 2007b).

This redefinition of mother support from a woman's and rights' perspective is a revolutionary break from traditional mother support group practices, which may in themselves be empowering to women, but are never articulated nor recognized as such. In fact, in 2005 during the 15 year review meeting of the Innocenti Declaration, WABA and its core partners advocated for the new The Innocenti Declaration 2005 to call for All Parties to "empower women in their own right, and as mothers and providers of breastfeeding support and information to other women" (Innocenti +15, 2005). Positioning mother support in this new framework makes it a recognizable platform for dialogue and exchange with the women's and rights movements, hopefully increasing opportunity for advocacy on the GIMS. From an advocacy point of view, it was hoped that the Initiative would help the breastfeeding movement link more broadly with natural childbirth and parenting groups, as well as women's health organizations that focus on women's reproductive health. Although the breastfeeding movement cannot provide all kinds of support, it can recognize the need for it, and whenever possible make efforts to link with other movements struggling for other support measures.

Three Key Outcomes of the LLLI/WABA State of the Art of Mother Support Summit

Following the well-coordinated online consultative dialogue process and the actual conference itself, the outcomes of the Mother Support Summit were specific and thus significant. The main outcome—which was a key response to question 4 of the dialogue—was a proposal to organize the 2008 WBW theme on Mother Support, as it would provide a global opportunity for thousands of individuals and groups to rally around a common cause at the same time. This activity aimed to increase visibility, support, and resources for Mother Support. The second outcome was to develop an interactive Mother Support Map on the Internet for easy and quick location of mother support resources worldwide; and the third, to produce a document of mother support text extracted from international documents to give greater legitimacy and authority to Mother Support and to position it as an element of international significance. A fourth and auxiliary outcome was the endorsement of the GIMS+5 Statement (Figure 11.1) by all the conference participants and a commitment to promote the GIMS endorsement far and wide, also with the intention of influencing policy change at the national level. This would work hand in hand with the third outcome of having a Mother Support document with international policy references. Finally, two additional recommendations were made: one to build the youth group as a sector for Mother Support, and secondly to strengthen the Fathers' and Men's Initiative.

The WABA Steering Committee approved the theme of mother support for the 2008 World Breastfeeding Week. Since 2008 was the year of the Olympics, it was decided that the WBW theme would be on "Mother Support: Going for the Gold," capitalizing on the idea of breastfeeding as the gold standard. When a child is breastfed, the family and the community is securing a winner! For WBW 2008, gold represents the best effort an individual or entity can make in supporting breastfeeding women. The word "gold" raises awareness of the superiority and the normalcy of breastfeeding. In 1997, breastfeeding had been declared the Gold Standard of Infant Feeding. Exclusive breastfeeding is the optimal food and feeding method for the first six months for the human infant, and it is the standard against which all other feeding methods must be measured. *We all win when babies are breastfed!*

The WBW 2008 theme content expanded on the diverse support systems a woman requires. WABA used the official OLYMPICS symbol of five interlocking colored rings for describing five CIRCLES OF SUPPORT for breastfeeding (see Chapter 1). These circles illustrate the potential influences on a mother's decision to breastfeed and to have a positive breastfeeding experience. The CIRCLES OF SUPPORT are: Family and Social Network, Healthcare, Government, Work and Employment, and Crisis and Emergency Situations, all surrounding the mother in the center circle. The objectives of this WBW campaign were:

- To expand awareness of the need for and the value of providing support to a breastfeeding mother.

- To disseminate updated information about support for breastfeeding mothers.

- To create optimal conditions for the provision of mother support in all CIRCLES OF SUPPORT.

In all, 541 groups reported participating in the WBW 2008 campaign. This involved more than 119,000 people in 100 countries. The theme also lent itself nicely to the following year's theme on emergencies and the need to support women in these especially difficult circumstances: natural disasters, refugee camps, divorce proceedings, critical illness of mother or baby, or living in an area of high HIV/AIDS prevalence with no support for breastfeeding.

The second outcome of the Summit was to develop an electronic map of mother support groups and contacts recognizable around the world. Never before has the world had such a listing of contacts that could be used and referred to by mothers and others in reaching mother support groups or resources. WABA launched the e-map in June 2009 and continues to invite people to indicate if they are mother support contacts (Figure 11.1). There are contacts listed in all regions of the world. Although from a global scale, many more mother support resources are needed in the Africa region.

A booklet with the long title, *Mother Support for Breastfeeding: Selected Statements and Excerpts about Mother Support in Key International Documents*, was produced in 2009 with the involvement of LLLI, and widely disseminated throughout the WABA network (Vickers, 2009). It is the first mother support resource for global advocacy, especially with the UN and other international agencies, and is a valuable resource for anyone who supports and protects breastfeeding. The booklet is formatted along the lines of the five circles of support from the 2008 WBW Action Folder, with the mother in the center. Each document, statement, or official text was charted and text included according to these five areas of support.

Today: Where Is the Global Movement on Mother Support?

Women will always need support for breastfeeding at a lesser or greater degree, depending on many general factors and each woman's specific situation. WABA and the WABA Mother Support Task Force are committed to continuing the efforts and activities that facilitate and broaden support for women around the world. The BFHI Step 10, even though limited in its scope, encourages support for a woman who has made the decision to breastfeed. Through WABA and the WABA Mother Support Task Force (MSTF), women are increasingly finding this support.

The *MSTF e-Newsletter* continues to be the major vehicle through which WABA promotes mother support. Although in 2011 the MSTF e-Newsletter was decreased from three issues a year to two issues, its importance to breastfeeding and mother support continues as strong as when it began in 2003. In 2011 the *e-Newsletter* first came out in Arabic and the possibility of a Chinese translation was seriously considered. Through the vehicle of the *e-Newsletter*, the GIMS is consistently promoted and endorsements secured, the Mother Support e-Map is promoted, and readers are invited to share their information.

In the past couple of years, WABA and the Mother Support Task Force have been promoting peer support and peer counselor training. There is increasingly compelling evidence that "peer support" is effective in supporting women to breastfeed. The Breastfeeding Gateway website provides a listing of current research articles and references in the section, "We're Here for You—Mother and Peer Support" (Figure 11.1). In countries where peer counseling has been funded and scaled up, breastfeeding rates have actually increased. While scaling up peer counseling requires more resources and the commitment of the public health system, WABA has started to support national training efforts, where feasible. This includes global advocacy to raise political support for this type of support intervention. All this is being done in an effort to increase the support that is needed by mothers all over the world.

Conclusion

The point of this chapter is to demonstrate that broader mother support efforts have been on-going globally over the past 20 years, almost simultaneously with the BFHI and the promotion of Step 10, in particular. While there is a strong need for the BFHI and Step 10, this chapter has made it clear that there is much more a woman needs for successful breastfeeding, which the BFHI and Step 10 alone cannot provide. Mother support needs to be broadened to ensure more holistic and comprehensive support that is respectful and sensitive to all women. WABA, with support from other breastfeeding organizations, continues to advocate for such broad measures by promoting the GIMS worldwide. If you are not already a GIMS+5 endorser, you should be one now! To become a GIMS+5 endorser, please visit http://www.waba.org.my/whatwedo/gims/gimsendorsement.htm.

Chapter Twelve

Supporting Mothers of Infants in the NICU

Beverly Rossman, PhD, RN
Michelle M. Greene, PhD
Amanda Kratovil, RN, BSN
Paula P. Meier, DNSc, RN, FAAN

INTRODUCTION

Human milk feedings are especially important for infants that are hospitalized in the neonatal intensive care unit (NICU) and for their mothers. For infants, human milk feedings program a myriad of body systems, thus impacting both short- and long-term health outcomes in this vulnerable population. For mothers, providing milk is often the only way they can continue to nurture and influence the health of their infants. This is especially important when all other caretaking activities have been assumed by professional caregivers in the NICU (Kavanaugh, Meier, Zimmerman, & Mead, 1997; Rossman et al., 2011). This chapter will outline the unique role of human milk feedings in reducing the risk of multiple costly and handicapping morbidities, integrate the provision of milk into the mother's coping with the NICU experience, introduce the Rush Mothers' Milk Club (RMMC), and end with a focus on mother support with examples from the RMMC.

Human Milk Feedings and Improved Outcome among NICU Infants

The unique nutritional, immunologic, growth-promoting, bioactive, and epigenetic components in human milk provide a species-specific form of protection for premature and sick newborns that are cared for in the NICU (Gartner et al., 2005; Meier, Engstrom, Patel, Jegier, & Bruns, 2010). In comparison to formula, human milk feedings facilitate the growth, maturation, and protection of the gastrointestinal tract, the brain, and other body organs. Additionally, human milk feedings received during the NICU hospitalization reduce the risk of late-onset sepsis, necrotizing enterocolitis, chronic lung disease, feeding intolerance, retinopathy of prematurity, and post-discharge complications in premature infants (Furman et al., 2004; Hylander, Strobino, & Dhanireddy, 1998; Hylander, Strombino, Pezzullo, & Dhanireddy, 2001; Meinzen-Derr et al., 2009; Schanler, Lau, Hurst, & Smith, 2005; Schanler, Shulman, & Lau, 1999; Uraizee & Gross, 1989; Vohr et al., 2006). These morbidities are costly, handicapping, and predisposing the affected infant to life-long health and educational problems. The role of human milk in reducing the risk of these complications and the best NICU practices to improve the use of human milk have been extensively reviewed in a recent publication (Meier et al., 2010).

Providing Human Milk as a Strategy for Maternal Helplessness and Passivity

Having an infant admitted to the NICU has been referred to as a "nightmare situation" for mothers (Charchuk & Simpson, 2005). Not only are mothers separated from their infants for at least some of the NICU hospitalization, but they must also cope with the inevitable stress and anxiety related to uncertainties about their infant's compromised medical status (Flacking, Ewald, Nyqvist, & Starrin, 2006; Johnson, 2008). Parents must also confront the machines and equipment required to provide intensive care for their critically ill infants. Mothers report being stressed by the sights and sounds of the NICU environment and the equipment, which may almost completely surround their baby (Miles, Burchinal, Holditch-Davis, Brunssen, & Wilson, 2002). All of these NICU "routines" make the environment emotionally challenging for families, and fuels a sense of helplessness with respect to doing anything to affect the infant's outcome. Several studies document the fact that mothers often feel intimidated by the expertise they witness from NICU nurses and assume a passive role in their infant's care as a result (Cleveland, 2008; Fenwick, Barclay, & Schmied, 2001; Heermann, Wilson, & Wilhelm, 2005; Lupton & Fenwick, 2001). Providing milk for a NICU infant and giving the mother as much control as possible over the processes of expression and feeding the milk have been proposed as strategies to reverse this sense of helplessness and passivity (Nyqvist & Engvall, 2009; Rossman et al., 2011).

Although the health outcomes of human milk feedings for NICU infants and their mothers are documented, mothers of infants hospitalized in the NICU typically encounter numerous barriers and challenges to the initiation and maintenance of lactation that are not experienced by mothers of healthy term infants (Callen & Pinelli, 2005). As a result, several studies show that these mothers, most of whom must initiate and maintain lactation with a breast pump, tend to experience problems with milk volume that are either temporary (delayed onset of lactation) or protracted (Cregan, De Mello, Kershaw, McDougall, & Hartmann, 2002; Hill, Aldag, Chatterton, & Zinaman, 2005a, 2005b). An array of well-documented barriers for successful provision of milk in the NICU have been described including: conflicting advice about the importance of human milk, selecting and using an appropriate breast pump, collecting and storing milk, and mothers observing clinicians treat their infant's slow weight gain with formula, even when the mother has an abundant supply of available milk (as reviewed in Meier et al., 2010). Addressing these barriers within the context of the NICU is complex because lactation care for these mothers requires advanced lactation knowledge and skills and is labor-intensive and time-consuming. Although lactation professionals often have experiences and education relevant to assisting mothers with breastfeeding healthy term infants and bedside NICU nurses can be supportive, neither may have the in-depth lactation expertise that the mothers need (Meier et al., 2010; Meier & Engstrom, 2007; Meier et al., 1993).

The culture of the NICU is unique; mothers of NICU infants have very different experiences than mothers of infants who are discharged home after birth (Meier et al., 2010; Padovani, Linhares, Pinto, Duarte, & Martinez, 2008; Punthmatharith, Buddharat, & Kamlangdee, 2007). The Rush Mothers' Milk Club is an exemplar of a program that removes lactation barriers for mothers of NICU infants. The RMMC is an evidenced-based lactation program that empowers mothers to provide their milk for their hospitalized NICU infants through sharing the science of human milk and lactation (www.rushmothersmilkclub.com). A unique feature of the RMMC is the inclusion of breastfeeding peer counselors (BPCs), all of whom were parents of a hospitalized NICU infant, as direct lactation care providers. The BPCs create an empowering environment for the parents by teaching them to perform independent creamatocrits on their milk and pre and post test-weights, thus allowing the parents, particularly the mothers to feel like the experts about their milk. This is an important psychological benefit, as it may help mothers persevere through the challenging and often frustrating or discouraging efforts associated with long-term pumping (Rossman et al., 2011).

RUSH MOTHERS' MILK CLUB (RMMC)

An exemplar of NICU mother-to-mother support is the RMMC, a program of evidence-based lactation care and human milk feedings in the 57-bed level III NICU at Rush University Medical Center. The RMMC has effectively adapted research on the effectiveness of peer breastfeeding support for low-income and ethnic minority mothers of term infants to the needs of mothers with NICU babies. Although it is not the primary topic of this chapter, the background research on the practice of BPCs with healthy, but vulnerable breastfeeding populations is summarized briefly in order to appreciate its adaptation to the NICU infant and mother.

The impact of BPCs on breastfeeding rates was first described by Kistin, Abramson, and Dublin (1994), and the data have consistently demonstrated the effectiveness of this role with vulnerable population groups of low-income, ethnic-minority mothers with healthy term infants (Anderson, Damio, Young, Chapman, & Perez-Escamilla, 2005; Arlotti, Cottrell, Lee, & Curtin, 1998; Chapman, Damio, Young, & Perez-Escamilla, 2004; Kistin et al., 1994; Long, Funk-Archuleta, Geiger, Mozar, & Heins, 1995; Schafer, Vogel, Viegas, & Hausafus, 1998; Shaw & Kaczorowski, 1999). Mothers of full-term infants who work with BPCs report fewer breastfeeding problems, greater satisfaction with the breastfeeding process, and appreciation of the increased social support that BPCs provide (Dennis, Hodnett, Gallop, & Chalmers, 2002; Locklin, 1995; Martens, 2002; Raine, 2003). The influence of BPCs on breastfeeding rates stems from their ability to support mothers, to motivate them to confront and challenge barriers to breastfeeding, and to persevere despite problems (Anderson et al., 2005; Chapman et al., 2004; Kistin et al., 1994). However, the definition of peer in these studies has been based almost exclusively on race, income, or community of residence (Anderson et al., 2005; Long et al., 1995; Martens, 2002; Schafer et al., 1998). In contrast, the RMMC conceptualizes the peer relationship as having experienced the birth, hospitalization, and the provision of human milk for an infant in the NICU (see Table 12.1). The "community" is the NICU environment, with its own unique set of challenges to the successful initiation and maintenance of lactation. The BPC, who represents this NICU community, serves as the experienced mother who shares her personal challenges, successes, and unique support mechanisms with respect to providing milk for an infant in the NICU. In a recent study, mothers valued this combination of attributes and indicated that the shared experience of having an infant in the NICU was at the heart of the BPC-new mother relationship, rather than any demographic similarity (Rossman et al., 2011).

Table 12.1. Breastfeeding Peer Counselors—Community vs NICU

Community Peer Counselors	NICU Peer Counselors
Shared experience between mothers and peer counselors based on demographics:	Shared experience between mothers and peer counselors based on being in the NICU:
Community of Residence Urban Rural	**NICU Community** Hospitalization of an infant Sharing with someone who's been through it
Socioeconomic Status Low Income WIC Eligible	**Long-Term Pumping** Providing Milk
Race/Ethnicity African American Hispanic Native American	**Separation from Infant** Coping with stress and anxiety related to infant's health status
	Using Lactation Technologies Creamatocrit Test weights Nipple Shields

Rush Mothers' Milk Club: An Overview

The RMMC is a comprehensive, empirically based program of interventions uniquely designed to promote and optimize the feeding of human milk for infants hospitalized in the NICU (Meier, Engstrom, Mingolelli, Miracle, & Kiesling, 2004). The RMMC is comprised of and defined by four major tenets: 1) sharing the science of human milk and lactation through communication and education, 2) use of evidence-based technology and resources, 3) removing barriers and improving accessibility to low-income and African-American mothers, and 4) integration of BPCs as primary lactation care providers (Meier et al., 2004; Meier et al., 2010).

SHARING THE SCIENCE OF HUMAN MILK AND LACTATION

The RMMC provides a framework for parent-NICU staff communication and education about providing human milk. Research about mothers of very low birth weight (VLBW; birthweight <1500g) infants reveals that direct, empirically supported conversations with a nurse or physician about providing human milk are not viewed as coercive by mothers and have a positive influence on their decision to provide their milk (Miracle, Meier, & Bennett, 2004). As such, within RMMC guidelines, families of NICU infants receive a consistent message that mother's milk is "medicine" for their infants that reduces the risk of complications of prematurity (Meier et al., 2010). Further, given the empirical support of human milk and the importance of communication, the RMMC ensures that NICU staff routinely supports mothers in providing milk regardless of the staff members' own personal opinions or beliefs (e.g., "I formula-fed my babies, and they are just fine.") (Meier et al., 2004; 2010). Other support that the RMMC provides includes educational material in a variety of media, including a series of written documents (e.g., packets and handouts) and a video that summarizes the benefits of mother's milk in a parent-and family-friendly, culturally sensitive manner ("In Your Hands," available at www. rushmothersmilkclub.com; Meier et al., 2004; Meier et al., 2010; Rush Mothers' Milk Club, n.d.).

EVIDENCE-BASED LACTATION TECHNOLOGY AND RESOURCES

Mothers' milk expression is supported by the RMMC's program of translational research, which incorporates evidence-based lactation technology for the routine management of human milk feedings and the transition to at-breast feeding for NICU infants and their families. For example, nipple shields, test-weights, and creamatocrits, which have been found to decrease the use of human milk alternatives, are integrated into mothers' NICU experiences (Meier et al., 2006; Meier et al., 2010).

The RMMC provides empirically-based expert consultation to mothers in two separate but complementary environments—at the mother's and infant's bedsides and at RMMC Luncheons. At the bedside, the BPCs meet with mothers and share evidence-based techniques to optimize milk output, feed infants at-breast, use lactation technology, and address common misconceptions about lactation and human milk on the part of friends and healthcare providers (Meier et al., 2004; Meier et al., 2010). The RMMC Luncheons provide NICU mothers with a nutritious free lunch that is part scientific discussion and part support group. Luncheons are attended by BPCs, NICU nurse lactation consultants, and the lactation program coordinator. All mothers with an infant hospitalized in or once hospitalized in the NICU are invited to attend this open group. Easy accessibility to staff in this informal setting, alongside peers and BPCs, provides mothers with yet another avenue for support in the NICU environment. Recently, RMMC has created a teaching video so other institutions can implement this group forum. Entitled "Lunch with the Rush Mothers' Milk Club: Sharing Science and Support," the video features an actual RMMC

Luncheon and highlights the empirical basis and social support of this forum (www.rushmothersmilkclub.com).

REMOVING LACTATION BARRIERS SPECIFIC TO LOW-INCOME AND AFRICAN-AMERICAN MOTHERS

African-American women are more than three times as likely as Caucasian or Hispanic women to give birth to a VLBW infant, are more than twice as likely to have that infant die within the first year of life, and yet are less likely than their Caucasian and Hispanic counterparts to provide milk for their infants (Centers for Disease Control and Prevention, 2011; Li & Grummer-Strawn, 2002). These differences highlight the importance of supporting low-income and African-American mothers by removing barriers to providing milk (Li & Grummer-Strawn, 2002). As such, the RMMC has subsequently created targeted interventions to provide lactation and social support for low-income and African-American mothers, including access to effective lactation equipment, information, and support.

A crucial step in developing and protecting an adequate volume of milk is the establishment of pumping with a hospital-grade electric breast pump, with a double collection kit, as soon after birth as possible (Hill, Aldag, & Chatterton, 2001; Hurst, Myatt, & Schanler, 1998; Meier et al., 2004; Spatz, 2004). Accessing double-setup electric breast pumps, however, is often difficult or impossible for low-income women, because purchasing or renting a pump is not economically feasible and public and private insurance companies may deny reimbursement (Chamberlain, McMahon, Philipp, & Merewood, 2006). The RMMC provides all mothers with hospital-grade electric breast pumps for use in the hospital and at home as needed. Additionally, immediately upon birth or transfer of the infant to the NICU, the RMMC provides mothers with milk storage containers and an insulated bag for safely transporting milk to the NICU (Meier et al., 2004).

The "Milk Club Taxi" is another important initiative in achieving access to information and support for low-income women. In order to reduce barriers to attending RMMC Luncheons (e.g., lack of transportation), mothers are offered free transportation to and from the luncheons through the RMMC Taxi. The RMMC Taxi service is well known throughout the NICU, and nurses and BPCs ensure that interested mothers are connected with this service.

INTEGRATION OF BPCs AS PRIMARY LACTATION CARE PROVIDERS

Since its inception in 1997, the RMMC has provided peer or mother-to-mother support to all mothers with an infant hospitalized in the Rush NICU. Initially, the peer support was provided by volunteer BPCs, who were the parents of former Rush NICU infants. The volunteer BPCs attended weekly RMMC luncheons, shared their stories and testimonies, and served as role models for other women. The BPCs also made follow-up phone calls and home visits to the mothers after their infants were discharged from the NICU as needed (Meier et al., 2004). Over time, the BPC role has expanded to its current status in which employed BPCs are available in the NICU every day of the week from approximately 7:00 a.m. until 9:00 p.m. for one-on-one care with new mothers. Every mother also has access to a pager, so they can reach a member of the lactation team at any time day or night.

BREASTFEEDING PEER COUNSELORS: FROM VOLUNTEER TO A PAID MEMBER OF THE NICU TEAM

Breastfeeding Peer Counselor education and scope of practice:

Each BPC completes a training course sponsored by La Leche League International to become a BPC. Upon being employed in the NICU, the BPC complete an additional three-month orientation program that provides them with specialized knowledge and skills for NICU lactation care. Throughout the orientation period, the BPC must successfully demonstrate that he or she can perform the appropriate lactation assessments and skills needed for NICU lactation practice.[6] The lactation practice model that has evolved features the BPCs working collaboratively and in consultation with the bedside neonatal nurse. The NICU lactation team

---

6   The BPCs have included a male as a valued member of the team. As the father of a baby who was born prematurely and a strong advocate for mother's milk, he was able to develop rapport with fathers, as well as assisting with other responsibilities.

includes nurse lactation specialists that are available for complicated scenarios that are beyond the scope of practice for the BPCs.

Other responsibilities that are assumed by the BPCs include visits to mothers that are hospitalized in the high-risk antepartum setting, consultation for lactation problems in the Pediatrics inpatient setting, all human milk storage management, and post-discharge NICU home visits. In addition, all BPCs serve as research assistants on externally funded research projects in the NICU. Selected BPCs assume an active role in lactation promotion activities at the city and state levels. The BPCs responsibilities are listed in Table 12.2.

Table 12.2. Peer Counselor Responsibilities

1. Introduction to Providing Milk
Introduce Rush Mothers' Milk Club to women in the antepartum unit
Within 24 hours contact each new mother whose infant is admitted to the NICU
2. Explain and Demonstrate Breast Pump Use and Milk Storage
Secure appropriate hospital grade electric pumps for mothers
Educate mothers about use of breast pump (frequency and duration)
Explain and demonstrate proper techniques for milk collection and storage
Teach mothers to collect, label, store and transport milk to the NICU
3. Protect Maternal Milk Volume
Implement the "Coming to Volume" Assessment Tool in first 14 days post-birth
Explain and demonstrate use of My Mom Pumps for Me! milk volume diaries
Conduct daily checks of the fit of breastshields during the NICU hospitalization
4. Assist with Transition Home from NICU
Teach mothers how to use breastpumps in the home
Participate in discharge planning to facilitate breastfeeding after NICU discharge

5. Maintain and Manage Lactation Programming
Participate in weekly Mother's Milk Club meetings
Assist in the management of the Women & Children's Nursing Breast Pump Rental Program
Maintain the human milk storage program for NICU infants

6. Involvement with Research and Advocacy
Participate in data collection and entry for research projects in the NICU
Act as a liaison between the Rush Mothers' Milk Club and local, regional, and national breastfeeding organizations

As the Rush BPCs become experienced and comfortable with their lactation care, they are individually mentored into assuming additional responsibilities. In fact, six Rush BPCs who began their employment as former parents have since become IBCLC-certified, and all BPCs assume responsibility for many interventions that are customarily performed by professional staff members, such as lactation consultants and NICU nurses. Thus, the RMMC BPC practice model includes both decision-making and technical assistance, and includes trouble-shooting such problems as inadequate maternal milk volume and performing creamatocrits and test-weights. The Rush BPC role is unique from other BPC roles in that it is hospital-based, highly specialized, and substitutive rather than additive with respect to professional lactation care providers. The BPCs perform approximately 75% of the lactation care in the NICU (Meier et al., 2010).

MOTHER-TO-MOTHER SUPPORT IN THE RUSH MOTHERS' MILK CLUB

Findings from a recent study of the Rush BPCs reveal that mothers were very accepting of the expanded BPC role, and perceived the BPCs as knowledgeable, competent, and caring (Rossman et al., 2011). These findings suggest that many of the lactation care responsibilities routinely assumed by lactation consultants and other NICU professionals can be provided by NICU BPCs, without compromising consumer satisfaction. In fact, findings indicate that many of the women preferred the BPC to the professional, primarily because the BPC had lived their experience and could support them in a culturally (i.e., NICU-specific) sensitive manner (Rossman et al., 2011). Three major conclusions on the part of the mothers reflect mother-to-mother support by the RMMC BPCs:

- The shared experience of having an infant in the NICU forms the basis of the relationship between the mother and the BPC and serves as a powerful motivator to initiate lactation, even if the mother has not planned to breastfeed.

- The BPCs provide the new mothers with information, assistance, and support to help them confront their own unique challenges to long-term breast pump dependency.

- The mothers find hope in their situations and feel empowered in their pumping and breastfeeding experiences by the BPCs' creation of an environment that facilitates meaningful and positive patterns of maternal-infant interactions.

The Shared Experience

The Rush BPCs are able to directly impact NICU lactation initiation and duration rates through the relationship they develop with the mothers. The BPCs share their stories of providing milk for their own infants when they were hospitalized in the NICU through pictures of their premature infants in the NICU and as growing and thriving children. They also include details of their infant's birth weight, gestational age, complications, and why they chose to provide their milk. The new mothers find hope in listening to the BPCs' stories and are encouraged about their own child's prospects when they learn that the BPC's infant may have been even less mature, smaller, or have experienced more complications than their own infant.

Many of the mothers and infants cared for in the RMMC are African-American and low-income, characteristics of women in the United States who are least likely to initiate lactation, but most likely to give birth to a VLBW infant (Centers for Disease Control and Prevention, 2006; MacDorman, Martin, Mathews, Hoyert, & Ventura, 2005). Some of the RMMC BPCs share this background and are especially credible when they serve as role models for this vulnerable, at-risk population. Many mothers of hospitalized NICU infants planned to formula feed at the time of their infant's birth, but changed their minds and persevered with providing milk after hearing the BPC's story of her own decision to change from formula to human milk. At-risk mothers relate their dedication to pumping to the BPC's ability to provide information and support to help them confront challenges to providing milk whenever a problem arises. Together, the mothers and BPCs form solutions that the mothers are comfortable with and can incorporate into their lifestyle. The importance of this connection between the BPC and the new mother, combined with the BPCs' creation of an empowering environment, appear to be powerful motivators for facilitating the initiation and duration of lactation in this population and supersedes relationships based on demographics (Rossman et al., 2011).

PEER COUNSELORS AND INFORMATION, ASSISTANCE, AND SUPPORT

During the initial visit by the BPC, the mother is given parent-focused information packets and handouts that translate the scientific principles about human milk and lactation into understandable words and concepts (Rush Mothers' Milk Club, 2008). The BPCs tell the mothers that providing their milk will help protect their NICU infant from many complications during and after their hospital stay. Since some mothers are unsure whether they want to feed their infants directly from their breast, the BPCs stress that the rewards of providing milk do not have to include the eventual feeding of the infant at their breast. Instead, they talk with the mothers about initially providing milk for a limited period of time to "get the baby off to the best start" (Meier et al., 2010). The BPCs will then reassure the mothers that all decisions about how long to pump and whether to feed at the breast can be made later in their infant's hospital stay.

Although there is an emphasis on the use of lactation technologies in the NICU to manage human milk feedings, BPCs help to "normalize the experience" for the mothers by helping them understand the personal relevance of providing milk for their infants. The BPCs bring each mother a hospital-grade electric breast pump and teach them the correct way to use and clean it. They observe the first few pumpings to ensure that the mother is using the pump correctly, help adjust the pump pressure, and custom fit the breast shields. Individualized pumping plans created together with the mother encourage the mother to persist, despite the many personal, emotional, or physical challenges that often arise when a mother is engaged in long-term milk expression.

The BPCs routinely employ the use of other lactation technologies, such as creamatocrits, to measure the lipid and calories in pumped milk, test weights, to accurately and precisely measure milk intake during breastfeeding of NICU infants, and nipple shields during the transition to feeding at-breast for premature infants. These technologies are standard care for managing lactation and human milk feeding in the Rush NICU. They can be performed by the BPCs, or they can be taught to mothers, so they can perform them independently (Meier et al., 2010). Contrary to some NICU health professional's opinions that these technologies may undermine a mother's confidence, several studies demonstrate that mothers appreciate and value the information provided by the procedure (Hurst, Meier, Engstrom, & Wyatt, 2004; Meier et al., 2010).

Prioritizing milk volume is one of the most important lactation responsibilities for the BPCs because an adequate milk volume is essential for exclusive human milk feedings and optimal transition to at-breast feedings (Meier et al., 2010). This is accomplished by teaching the mothers to monitor how much milk they pump using the "My Mom Pumps For Me!" log book. Together, the mother and BPC set individualized measurable milk volume targets. The BPCs are then able to track a mother's milk volume through daily monitoring with the "Coming to Volume" checklist (Rush Mothers' Milk Club, 2008) and are able to identify and help manage low volume in the early stages. This empowering environment created by the BPCs helps the mothers to experience a sense of pride in witnessing the results of providing milk and doing what only they can do to make their babies healthy, and grow and thrive (Rossman et al., 2011).

"Mothering the Mother"

The NICU-based BPCs also help promote maternal confidence by creating an environment that facilitates meaningful and positive patterns of maternal-infant interactions (Rossman et al., 2011). When an infant is admitted to the NICU, the maternal role evolves in a public, medically focused context, with limited caretaking opportunities. Mothers often feel inadequately prepared to care for their child and may be overwhelmed with stress and feelings of depression and guilt (Black, Holditch-Davis, & Miles, 2009; Emmanuel, Creedy, St. John, & Brown, 2011; Holditch-Davis & Miles, 2000; Lupton & Fenwick, 2001; Reid, 2000; Shin & White-Traut, 2007). The BPCs often use chatting as a clinical tool to provide emotional support for mothers and to facilitate confidence in the mothering role. Chatting is a type of everyday communication that minimizes the power differential and invites two-way conversations as a way of reaching women on a personal and emotional level (Fenwick et al., 2001). This informal communication demonstrates to the mothers that the BPCs care for and about them. Creation of such an emotionally supportive and protective environment is often referred to as "mothering the mother" (Klaus, Kennell, & Klaus, 1993). In an anthropological study on breastfeeding, Raphael (1981) noted that the one element in most cultures which facilitated success in breastfeeding was the presence of someone who dedicated their care to the mother. In the Rush NICU, this person is the BPC. Mothers feel nurtured and cared for as the BPCs communicate in a manner that conveys compassion for the mother's experience, and acknowledge and respond to their concerns (Dennis, 2002; Morrow et al., 1999; Mozingo, Davis,

Droppleman, & Merideth, 2000; Nelson, 2006; Rossman et al., 2011). This type of rapport is important because the mothers perceive that the insights gained from these informal discussions help them establish, maintain, and enhance their confidence as a mother (Rossman et al., 2011). Through their interactions with the BPCs, mothers also recognize that providing milk goes beyond better health outcomes for their infants. Through the knowledge that providing milk is the one tangible contribution only they can make to their infants' health, mothers experience greater mother-infant attachment, as well as enhanced self-esteem (Bernaix, Schmidt, Jamerson, Seiter, & Smith, 2006; Callen & Pinelli, 2005; Flacking et al., 2006; Miracle et al., 2004). In addition, making a connection on an informal basis "with someone who actually dealt with it" helps to alleviate some of the social isolation, stress, and anxiety common to mothers with infants hospitalized in the NICU (Johnson, 2008; Jones, Woodhouse, & Rowe, 2007; Preyde & Ardal, 2003; Sisk, Lovelady, Dillard, Gruber, & O'Shea, 2009).

Summary

The RMMC is an evidenced-based lactation program that empowers mothers to provide their milk for their hospitalized NICU infants through sharing the science of human milk and lactation and removing barriers to lactation for vulnerable at-risk populations. Working collaboratively with the bedside NICU nurse, the BPCs provide mother-to-mother support and lactation care on a daily basis and share their personal experiences of the birth, hospitalization, and unique challenges of providing human milk for an infant in the NICU. By virtue of this shared experience, the BPCs are able to help mothers manage pumping and breastfeeding, as well as cope with the emotional stress of having an infant hospitalized in the NICU. Best practices to increase the rates of human milk feedings in other NICU settings should incorporate BPCs with personal experience of providing milk for a hospitalized infant.

Chapter Thirteen

Breastfeeding Support Groups for Mothers of Multiple-Birth Infants and Children

Karen Kerkhoff Gromada, MSN, RN, IBCLC, FILCA

INTRODUCTION

My Breastfeeding Twins Story

In March 1977 I gave birth to my third and fourth children within ten minutes. I was lucky to be among the fewer than 15% of women pregnant with twins—both then and now—who go into spontaneous labor at full term (40 weeks, 5 days), and the even fewer who have an unmedicated, vaginal delivery for both babies. Each breastfed within 45-90 minutes of birth, and we roomed in for 60 hours with no separation, but also little sleep for me, and then we all went home. Neither baby had anything other than my milk from birth until some point between six and seven months, when each began signaling an interest in complementary foods. Both gained more than two pounds (about a kilo) a month for their first several months. Each continued to breastfeed until sometime after his second birthday.

In spite of having breastfed two single-born children into toddlerhood and an "ideal" twins breastfeeding story, the four to five years of my twin pregnancy and the early mothering of infant and toddler twins are among the most physically and emotionally difficult years of my life. Prior experiences with two single-born children did not prepare me for the different dynamics of breastfeeding and caring for two same-age infants/children. I often felt completely overwhelmed, exhausted, and unsupported. In these aspects of twin pregnancy and mothering, I am among an evidence-based majority (Beck, 2002a).

My Breastfeeding Support System

I'd been a La Leche League (LLL) member for five years and a LLL Leader for two years when our twins were born. I'd had opportunities to watch women breastfeed twins before I found myself in this special situation. I knew twins could be exclusively breastfed; I'd seen it, and seeing helps believing.

My LLL co-leaders were incredibly supportive about breastfeeding twins, but their strategies for the logistical, "how-to" management of two high-need newborns, which I desperately needed, often lacked credibility for me. None of my co-leaders had breastfed twins. They'd never had to juggle two crying newborns, while also caring for two preschoolers. They hadn't dealt with two newborns who needed to breastfeed at the same time, yet also had difficulty latching. Their hearts weren't breaking when they couldn't meet the needs of two young infants who needed and deserved to be comforted by a mother who couldn't figure out how to meet both babies' needs at once. They simply couldn't know what it was like.

I wanted to try some of their suggestions, but I worried what would happen if a strategy made things worse instead of better. I often felt I was barely staying afloat both physically and mentally during those early months. I worried that if a strategy made life more difficult, I might go under. So I usually called a mother of twins (MOT) in the LLL group who was breastfeeding toddler boy/girl twins to get her opinion on suggestions offered by others or to check for twin-tested ideas.

I don't mean to minimize the importance of my co-leaders' support. In a culture that often undermines a woman's choice to breastfeed the single-born infant, support and belief in a mother's ability to nourish two or more multiple-birth infants is crucial. Plus, it is only thanks to one of my co-leaders that I was able to attend the LLL International (LLLI) conference with four-month-old twins. There I met many other Leaders who were breastfeeding or had breastfed twins, and I met the Leader who gave me the idea to start a mothers of multiples-only LLL group (MOM group) when she told me about the special meetings she held two or three times a year. Why stop with occasional meetings when women breastfeeding multiples needed to talk year round with others who'd breastfed multiples?

BIRTH OF A MULTIPLES-SPECIFIC BREASTFEEDING GROUP

To form a "special" LLL group for women breastfeeding twins or more, I had to submit paperwork to the LLLI office. Not a task I enjoyed at the time, it proved to be an important exercise. LLLI asked me to justify the request by documenting the need for a special Mothers of Twins/Mothers of Multiples (MOT/MOM) group versus attendance at "traditional" LLL group meetings. This better prepared me when I initially planned and facilitated group meetings. The submitted literature review reminded me that most of the mothers attending meetings and calling with breastfeeding questions would not have had the breastfeeding beginning I'd enjoyed with my twin sons.

The Cincinnati (Ohio, USA) LLL Multiples group received approval to meet and held its first meeting in September 1977 when my twins were six months. Another local MOT, who was also accredited as a LLL leader, agreed to be the group's co-leader. Since the group's inception, only women who have breastfed multiple-birth infants/children can serve as a Leader of this LLL multiples group.

One of the most valuable aspects of our special group has been the opportunity to distinguish breastfeeding and related mothering or family issues that are common or specific to breastfeeding multiple-birth infants/toddlers from those of a particular mother or family. As a breastfeeding support group "leader" of a group comprised completely of women breastfeeding multiple-birth infants and toddlers for more than 30 years, I've heard "my" story repeated many times, as well as in many variations. I am often in awe of the group mothers, many of whom have overcome incredible obstacles to breastfeed and provide their milk for their multiples.

Need for Specialized Information and Support

To provide appropriate information and support to women breastfeeding or expressing milk for multiple-birth infants, it is important to recognize that support is about much more than the "mechanics" of putting two, three, or more babies to breast. Although only 3% of births are multiple births, this number represents a doubling of multiple births in western nations since 1980, due mainly to increases in assisted reproductive technology (ART) (Martin et al., 2011; Australian Bureau of Statistics, 2010; Statistics Canada, 2009; D'Addato, 2007). In addition, today's MOT/MOM initiate breastfeeding or milk expression at rates approximating those of women pregnant with a single infant (Mothers of Supertwins [MOST], 2007; Östlund, Nordström, Dykes, & Flacking, 2010; Ooki, 2008; Yokoyama et al, 2006; Damato, Dowling, Standing, & Schuster, 2005). (Most research does not distinguish between direct breastfeeding and expressed-breastmilk-feeding [EBMF].) The number of women who exclusively breastfeed or EBMF twin multiples may be significantly lower than for those breastfeeding single-born infants (Yokoyama et al., 2006; Ooki, 2008), yet a drop in the number who continue some breastfeeding or EBMF follows a pattern similar to that of single-born infants (Damato, Dowling, Madigan, & Thanattherakul, 2005; Geraghty, Pinney, Sethurman, Roy-Chaudbury, & Kalkwarf, 2004). Not surprisingly, direct breastfeeding has been associated with improved duration of breastfeeding (Geraghty, Khoury, & Kalkwarf, 2005).

It's Complicated

A woman planning to breastfeed multiple newborns needs the best possible breastfeeding start, yet she and her babies are the least likely to get it. For many physiological and emotional reasons, each of her multiple babies deserve their mother's milk and the breastfeeding relationship as much as a single-born infant. However, name any maternal or newborn complication of pregnancy, labor, or birth, and one or more of them are significantly more likely to occur with multiples throughout pregnancy, birth, and the postnatal period. So, MOT/MOM must often establish lactation via milk expression followed by the eventual and individual transition of two, three, or more infants to direct breastfeeding, while also maintaining milk production via continued milk expression until both/all effectively breastfeed, or continue long-term EBMF for one or more of the babies. Neither alternative is a minor feat.

Infant-Related Issues

The most significant complication of multiple pregnancy is the increased likelihood of preterm or late preterm birth. Although the most recent birth data for the United States found multiple births accounted for only 3% of all births, they comprised 17% of all infants born prior to 37 weeks completed gestation and 23% of all births considered "very preterm," with birth prior to 32 weeks of gestation (Martin et al., 2010). Compared with 38.7 weeks as the average length of gestation (ALG) for a single-born infant, the ALG for twins was 35.3 weeks with decreasing ALG for each additional multiple. The EURO-PERISTAT Project (2008) reported similar statistics for European nations.

In addition, one or more of multiple-birth sets are several times more likely than the single-born to be affected by intrauterine growth restriction (IUGR) (Bowers & Gromada, 2006), with related low birth weight (LBW) of 5 lb, 8 oz/2500 gm or less, or very low birth weight (VLBW) of 3 lb, 3 oz/1500 gm or less, irrespective of a set's gestational age (Martin et al., 2010; EURO-PERISTAT Project, 2008). The greater the number of multiples in a set the greater is the likelihood of LBW and VLBW. Multiples, particularly monozygotic (MZ)/"identical" ones, are also at increased risk for congenital or pregnancy-related anomalies, and placental or umbilical cord deviations (Pharoah & Dundar, 2009; Glinianaia, Rankin, & Wright, 2008; Bowers & Gromada, 2006; Tang et al., 2006). Infant mortality for multiples is about five times that of single-birth infants (Mathews & MacDorman, 2010). The implications for maternal attachment formation, while also grieving for the multiple(s) that died can affect breastfeeding or milk expression for the survivor(s) (Gromada & Bowers, 2005; Pector, 2004; Hanrahan, 2000).

Finally, one or more of the multiples are more likely to be affected by related transient or chronic morbidities associated with preterm birth, LBW/VLBW, or an anomaly. These health conditions can result in ongoing post-discharge care visits that disrupt direct breastfeeding or milk expression, as the mother must choose whether to manage more than one baby in an outpatient setting, leave one or more infants at home, and then consider if it's possible and when/how to express milk while away from home.

Mother-Related Issues

An increased risk for maternal complications with multiples also contributes to delays in initiating breastfeeding or milk expression. According to Bowers and Gromada (2006), women pregnant with multiples are several times more likely to be affected by pregnancy-induced hypertension (PIH), sometimes referred to as pre-eclampsia or toxemia, and its more serious variation of HELLP (Hemolysis, Elevated Liver enzymes, Low Platelets). The incidence of gestational diabetes mellitus (GDM) increases 1.8 times with each additional multiple over that of a single-pregnancy. Anemia during pregnancy is two to three times higher among women pregnant with multiples. Perinatal hemorrhage, which occurs with 1.2% of single-infant pregnancies, affects 6% of twin, 12% of triplet, and 21% of quadruplet pregnancies, and is most often due to placental conditions or postnatal uterine atony.

In addition, the new mother of multiples may be twice or more as likely to be recovering postnatally from a surgical delivery (CDC, 2009) and the physical and emotional effects of strict prenatal bed rest (Maloni, 2010), while assuming the care of two or more newborns. Finally, certain health conditions that are also associated with ART to achieve pregnancy may also be associated with lower milk production (West & Marasco, 2008). Is it any wonder then that women giving birth to multiples are at several times more risk of developing a postpartum mood disorder (PPMD) (Choi, Bishal, & Minkovitz, 2009)?

OFFERING INFORMATION AND SUPPORT

The obstacles many new mothers face when initiating breastfeeding with multiple newborns can feel overwhelming at times. It is not necessary for leaders of support groups and health professionals to have breastfed multiples themselves in order to offer information, ideas, encouragement, and support to women breastfeeding or expressing milk for multiples. However, it is important that they *know they don't know*, as they are more apt then to seek appropriate, multiples-specific resources for these mothers and adapt strategies to fit the more complex physical and emotional management of breastfeeding and caring for two or more infants.

Prenatal Support

When working with a woman pregnant with multiples, obstetric care providers, their office or clinic staff, and group support leaders can achieve both Step 3 (antenatal breastfeeding education) and Step 10 of the *Ten Steps to Successful Breastfeeding* by promoting breastfeeding, encouraging pregnancy and birth behaviors more likely to result in no, or fewer, complications for mother and babies, and providing anticipatory guidance for establishing lactation and human-milk-feedings, whether or not initiation is affected by maternal or infant(s) complications. Strategies may include:

- Informing these women of the species-specific immunological, nutritional, and psychosocial properties found only in breastfeeding and human milk (Leonard, 2003).

- Treating each woman with a multiple pregnancy as the unique entity she—and it—is. One size of obstetrical care does NOT fit all multiple pregnancies or multiple births (Gromada, 2007).

- Encouraging adequate maternal weight gain, which has been associated with birth at greater gestational age and larger birth weights for multiples (Fox et al., 2010).

- Examining the breasts and assessing maternal history for any condition that may affect milk production (West & Marasco, 2008), while reassuring her that most women are capable of producing enough milk for two and even more infants (Saint, Maggiore, & Hartmann, 1986).

- Sharing supportive information specific to breastfeeding multiples, particularly stories of other women who breastfed and expressed milk for twins or more (Welsh, 2011; Szucs, Axline, & Rosenman, 2010; Szucs, Axline, & Rosenman, 2009; Berlin, 2007; Gromada, 2006; Leonard, 2000; Auer & Gromada, 1998; Mead, Chuffo, Lawlor-Klean, & Meier, 1992).

- Helping the expectant mother to develop a family-centered birth/early postpartum plan that accommodates vaginal or surgical delivery followed by initial breastfeeding for each healthy, stable term or late preterm multiple within 60-90 minutes of birth or the early initiation of milk expression if one or more newborns requires special care.

- Encouraging mother-babies rooming-in on the postpartum unit with round-the-clock rotation of a family member or friend acting as mother's helper, especially after surgical birth.

- Encouraging the expectant mother to formalize a breastfeeding plan by writing her short- and long-term goals for breastfeeding/lactation (Gromada, 2007).

- Referring the expectant mother to, and encouraging her to attend, local multiples-specific or general breastfeeding support group meetings and classes (Gromada, 2011a, b), and to make contact with breastfeeding mothers at local or regional parents/mothers of multiples groups.

- Encouraging the woman to build a breastfeeding support system. The list may include the woman's husband/partner, other women who have breastfed multiples, breastfeeding support group leaders, IBCLCs, and family and friends who will encourage the new mother of multiples to work through any initial bumps in the breastfeeding road.

- Encouraging the development of a plan for help with household tasks during the postnatal period, so the new mother is freer to get to know and breastfeed (or pump for) her babies (LLLI, 2009).

Intrapartum (Birth/Postnatal unit)

To best achieve Step 10, Labor and Delivery, Postnatal/Mother-Baby, and Newborn Intensive Care (NICU) units should begin by fulfilling the nine steps preceding it. In addition, it is important to assess and treat each multiple-birth newborn as an individual, while also acknowledging that each one's arrival as part of a set affects maternal (and others') behaviors and her/their approaches toward the babies by:

- Observing each term (or almost term) newborn breastfeed alone/separately.

- Encouraging rooming-in, so the mother may feed each newborn on cue.

- Suggesting a mother wait to feed two at once until at least one latches fairly easily and demonstrates effective breastfeeding behaviors. However, show her various positioning for simultaneous breastfeeding, so she has options when her babies are ready.

- Encouraging a mother to express her milk both manually and mechanically (Morton et al., 2009) if multiples are preterm and not yet able to transfer milk effectively during breastfeeding. Reinforce that it is important to express milk regularly even if she obtains only drops of colostrum in the first days. Let her know how valuable her milk is by collecting those drops via a syringe to give to babies.

- Reinforcing post-discharge multiples-specific or general breastfeeding support resources via phone and group meetings. In addition, inform the new mother that Internet information and support groups specifically established to support mothers breastfeeding twins or higher multiples are available online.

Postnatal Support

General Information

Community breastfeeding support groups or networks become crucial after hospital discharge when mothers of young multiples tend to feel most overwhelmed (Beck, 2002a). Group leaders can encourage a mother of multiples to:

- Review each of her goals for breastfeeding as often as needed, which often makes it easier for a mother to revise her route to reach a breastfeeding goal if she faces a breastfeeding "detour" along the way.

- Engage in kangaroo mother care with her babies separately or all together, whether the babies are in a NICU or at home.

- Revise any milk expression plan needed to provide milk for multiples in the NICU or any with ineffective breastfeeding behaviors. Rigid plans may not work for a particular mother. It is possible to "fit" adequate milk expression with her real life!

- Keep in mind that each baby in a multiples set is a unique individual with his/her own behavioral approach to breastfeeding. This means one preterm multiple is likely to be ready to transition to direct breastfeeding when another needs more time. Or one may do well with eight feedings, yet another may need more than 10 in 24 hours to gain weight and thrive. This is a difficult concept for mothers of multiples because many/most feel a competing desire to treat each multiple as separate, yet also treat them as equal (Beck, 2002b).

- Distinguish true breastfeeding issues from two (or more) babies' issues. The physical management and logistics when caring for two or more infants/toddlers night and day often results in questions or concerns that seem to be breastfeeding-related when they are not.

- Obtain needed household help. It is not realistic for a mother to think she can care for two or more infants/toddlers without more physical household help. Such help frees her to focus on breastfeeding her multiples and caring for them and any older children.

Nighttime Breastfeeding

Sleep deprivation is a profound and often long-term issue for many women caring for two or more same-age infants through toddlers. When significant maternal sleep deprivation affects her daytime behavior, all family members are affected. Yet nighttime strategies that promote both breastfeeding and better sleep for both a mother and her single infant, such as safe bedsharing techniques may not be as easy or as safe to implement with multiple infants, particularly if multiples were born preterm. The following suggestions may help:

- Be aware that a number of organizations for parents of multiples encourage so-called "sleep training" with multiple newborns, including the ignoring of infants' cries and the development of a (rigid) schedule in the name of parents' "survival." Breastfeeding support leaders provide a crucial service when they educate parents about infants' nighttime needs, variations in need for individual infants, and that crying is an infant's way to communicate distress. This information may require frequent repetition, as there are (many) nights when "sleep training" rhetoric may tempt sleep-deprived parents.

- Share with mothers that breastfed infants and mothers in close proximity to each other tend to develop more synchronous sleep state patterns (McKenna & Gettler, 2007), and recent studies associated exclusive breastfeeding with more maternal sleep and daytime energy (Kendall-Tackett, Cong, & Hale, 2011).

- Mothers have long reported their twins "slept better" when close together and sharing a single crib (cot). Research by Ball (2007) appears to reinforce this notion. She found that co-bedded twins demonstrated more synchronous sleep states without an increase in sleep-environment risk.

- Sleep solutions that are sensitive to both infants and their mother vary from family to family. Options may include:

1.   Bedsharing for all or part of the night in the parents' bed. Options have included the placing of a king-size or several different sizes of firm mattresses on the floor of the parents' room or a mattress in a "nursery" bedroom, which the mother moves to once one or more babies begin to wake for night feeding.

2.   Co-sleeping of infants in some form of a co-sleeper, often a crib (cot) near or attached to the parents' bed. Some co-sleeping mothers bedshare with one infant at a time, rotating infants in and out of the maternal/parental bed as one infant wakes to breastfeed. Other mothers prefer to get up for feedings. These mothers often try to wake the second baby to breastfeed with or immediately after the first multiple. (A mother of triplets may do both—wake a second to feed with the first and wake a third immediately afterward.)

3.   Getting help with feedings. To ensure that a mother gets a few hours of uninterrupted sleep, still other parents occasionally or regularly alternate a breastfeeding (or two) with a bottle-feeding of mother's milk or infant formula if mother's milk or human milk is unavailable. One parent may handle the feeding for both/all babies or a mother may breastfeed one while the helper feeds another. The ability to have occasional or regular help with infants' night feedings may influence the initiation or continuation of breastfeeding with multiples, yet support leaders should share potential implications. Mothers should understand that occasional help with feedings, which results in missing one or more breastfeedings, may contribute to plugged ducts or mastitis for breasts that have been producing for two, three, or more infants, and regular feeding help may result in decreased milk production.

Information/Support Group Meeting Logistics

A mother of multiples who would like to attend breastfeeding support group meetings may:

•   Attend meetings intermittently due to pregnancy bed rest, a concern about taking former preterm infants out during RSV (respiratory syncytial virus) season, and so on. Transporting and moving two or more infants to and from a meeting may seem worthwhile or overwhelming, depending on the weather.

•   Need help with transportation or to get into and out of group meetings. Evaluate a meeting location for accessibility and develop a way she may signal for help when needed, such as using a mobile phone to contact a group leader to come and help.

- Want group leaders or those attending without babies to provide extra arms to hold or soothe a multiple, but she may feel uncomfortable asking for this help. Observe and ask if you may hold a baby for her if she appears to need help.

- Need a (big) glass of water or a snack, but be unable to get up to obtain it.

- Feel embarrassed or uncomfortable if one or more infants are to be fed at meetings via an alternative feeding method, such as a tube device at breast or an infant feeding-bottle, or if one or more is exclusively human-milk-fed or given an artificial infant milk (AIM) rather than breastfed directly, no matter what the reason.

Group leaders may need to evaluate their thoughts and feelings as they pertain to the breastfeeding support group goals when a mother of multiples still depends on feeding bottles or artificial infant milk for one or more infants still transitioning to direct breastfeeding, or she has chosen to partially breastfeed multiples. Support group leaders should consider honestly their own level of comfort and ability to support mothers who bottle-feed one or more infants at a group meeting with expressed human milk or artificial infant milk. The thoughts or feelings of other mothers in attendance may also be a consideration. Anticipation and advance planning, such as through leader-to-leader role play, may be useful.

What to Do and Not Do

When you are working with a MOT/MOM:

- Don't say, "I know what you're going through," unless you've breastfed multiples yourself. (Even when someone has tandem-nursed two or more different-age nurslings, the experiences cannot compare since both/all of different-aged nurslings were likely born at term, at least one has more head/body control for self-positioning at breast, and their mother had an opportunity to form an attachment with one before repeating the experience with another.)

- Do let a mother of multiples know that you recognize you have not been in her situation and ask that she let you know if she thinks a helping strategy seems unrealistic or she feels uncertain or concerned about implementing it. And ask which aspects of the strategy seem unrealistic or cause concern, so they may be addressed or revised.

- Don't ask if she conceived her babies "naturally" or via fertility treatment. (She has been asked this many times.)

- Do network as needed to find another mother or a breastfeeding support leader who is breastfeeding a set of same-number multiples to share with the mother in case she would ever want to communicate with the other mother of multiples.

- Do "praise" the mother in the form of reinforcement, but don't point to her as the group "supermom" simply because she breastfeeds multiple-birth children!

CONCLUSION

That Was Then, This Is Now!

Cincinnati LLL Multiples continues to meet today, although the group has had to change with the times. MOT/MOM are different than they were at the group's inception. Today's mother of multiples is as likely, or more likely, to join an Internet mother-to-mother breastfeeding support (Figure 13.1) and information group as an in-person group. Participation in either has advantages and disadvantages and, fortunately, participation in one does not preclude participation in the other. When no in-person peer support is available, a mother of multiple's participation in both a local in-person breastfeeding mothers group and an online breastfeeding mothers of multiples support group may enhance the strengths of each.

This account explores my personal experience of establishing a multiples-specific mother-to-mother support group and the wider issue of the value of contact with true peers—women who have lived the experience of breastfeeding twins or higher multiples—and the special needs involved for both mothers and infants. It was to meet these needs that MOT/MOM in-person and Internet groups were set up. Finally, the suggestions in this chapter should be considered within the context of the *Ten Steps to Successful Breastfeeding* of the Baby-Friendly Hospital Initiative, especially Step 3 (breastfeeding education during pregnancy) and Step 10 (mother support).

Figure 13.1. Breastfeeding Multiples: Online Mother-To-Mother Support

APMultiples (Attachment Parenting Multiples) Yahoo Group: http://groups.yahoo.com/group/apmultiples/

Mothering Multiples: Breastfeeding and Caring for Twins or More—Facebook Page https://www.facebook.com/pages/Mothering-Multiples-Breastfeeding-and-Caring-for-Twins-or-More/248855546696?ref=ts

Parenting Multiples (Mothering.com Forum) http://www.mothering.com/community/f/158/parenting-multiples

Chapter Fourteen

Overcoming Barriers Through New Technology: Support Via Text Messaging

Rebekah Russell-Bennett (Queensland University of Technology)
Danielle Gallegos (Queensland University of Technology)
Josephine Previte (University of Queensland)

INTRODUCTION

Despite the significant health benefits attributed to breastfeeding, rates in countries such as Australia continue to remain static or to decline. Latest data from the Longitudinal Survey of Australian Children indicate that only 56% of infants at three months are fully breastfed, decreasing to 14% at six months (Australian Institute of Family Studies, 2008). Similar figures are reported in the United States, with exclusive breastfeeding rates at six months put at 14.8% (Center for Disease Control and Prevention, 2011). There are significant reductions in breastfeeding rates at one month of age, and again at four months (Australian Institute of Family Studies, 2008).

With access to mobile phone networks at 90 percent worldwide and with 110 subscriptions for every 100 people in Australia across all areas of advantage and disadvantage (World Bank, 2009), using mobile technology (m-technology) to change health behaviors is a viable mode of intervention. The MumBubConnect (MBC) program was developed by researchers in the social marketing and public health fields in conjunction with the Australian Breastfeeding Association (ABA) to investigate the use of technology as a support technique for new mothers to assist them in overcoming barriers to maintaining breastfeeding.

MumBubConnect is the world's first two-way automated Short-Message-Service (SMS) program that provides support for new breastfeeding mothers. The program was trialed in 2010 for eight weeks with 120 Australian women to test the technology and identify the effectiveness of text messaging in a social marketing program. Evaluation measures indicated that the program not only increased social support and self-efficacy, but was also highly valued by the women as an important resource for breastfeeding. This chapter provides details of the development and implementation of MumBubConnect, an innovative text messaging support program developed using strong public health and social marketing theoretical constructs.

PURPOSE/PHILOSOPHY

Organizations, governments, and health professionals use a variety of tools to change breastfeeding behavior, including changing public policy, reorienting health services, training of health professionals, education programs, and awareness/knowledge campaigns (Dyson et al., 2010; Fairbank, O'Meara, Renfrew, Snowden, & Lister-Sharp, 2000; Protheroe, Dyson, Renfrew, Bull, & Mulvihill, 2003). Awareness campaigns for breastfeeding typically position breastfeeding as a simple "doable" behavior, relying on "rosy images" that often deny the challenges that confront women. Increasingly, governments and other organizations are seeking economically viable ways to increase tangible support for women as they breastfeed. Prior research on the use of text messaging has shown positive results in influencing other health behaviors, but not specifically for breastfeeding.

Social marketing is the application of commercial marketing principles to address social issues, such as improving health, decreasing use of dangerous substances, and increasing environmentally-friendly practices (Kotler & Lee, 2008). Governments around the world are turning to social marketing as an intervention tool to improve social outcomes, as awareness campaigns and law enforcement fail to change behaviors. The key elements of social marketing that distinguish the approach from public health campaigns are the emphasis on the consumer, the notion of exchange (cost-benefit), identification of the competing factors for the desired behavior, and the application of the marketing mix (4Ps) (Rothschild, 1999). For any campaign to be considered social marketing, it needs to fulfill eight benchmarks established by the National Social Marketing Centre in the United Kingdom. These benchmarks as they apply to MumBubConnect are outlined in Figure 14.1.

Figure 14.1. Social Marketing Criteria

Applying Social Marketing to Breastfeeding

1. Consumer orientation: Places new mothers at the heart of the program and commences the program design from the realities identified by the recipients. MumBubConnect took a mother-oriented rather than a baby-oriented approach.

2. Behavior and behavioral goals: While attitudes are important, social marketing aims to influence behaviors. The behavior in new mothers that was targeted by MumBubConnect was continuation of any breastfeeding.

3. Theory: The underpinning theories used to design MumBubConnect were seeking-social-support coping theory (Vitaliano, Russo, Carr, Maiuro, & Becker, 1985) and self-efficacy (Bandura, 1977).

4. Consumer insight: Qualitative research was conducted as formative research to guide the project. This research identified that women found breastfeeding hard (it didn't come naturally), felt they had failed if they could not breastfeed, were confused by conflicting advice from the medical community, and wanted support that was non-intrusive, non-judgmental, and personalized. The research also identified that women liked the idea of receiving SMS (Short Message Service) as a means of breastfeeding support.

5. Exchange: The social costs (time, pain, energy, self-esteem) associated with breastfeeding were perceived as high compared to the benefits. When this imbalance increased as breastfeeding problems occurred, the value offered by breastfeeding diminished in favor of alternative feeding methods where the social cost was lower. MumBubConnect aimed to reduce the social cost by improving social support and self-efficacy.

6. Competition: The competition to breastfeeding could be the influence of other people (partner, family, friends), work requirements, availability of other feeding options (formula, water, food), and cultural values that privilege formula feeding. MumBubConnect aimed to combat competing messages and behaviors from other people by normalizing breastfeeding challenges and positively encouraging breastfeeding through text messages.

7. Marketing Mix: MumBubConnect adopted the 4 Ps of commercial marketing when designing the program:

- Product: A service delivered by Short Message Service with the Australian Breastfeeding Association provided outbound counseling calls in response to some texts, a website that offered advice and information, a social networking site, and wallet cards/refrigerator magnets with program details.
- Price: Both the financial cost of participating (free) and the social costs associated with the program (see point 5). The focus on any breastfeeding rather than exclusive breastfeeding reduced the social price of breastfeeding.
- Place: Relates to access to the product (service). The service was available 24/7, 24 hours a day via the mother's own phone, was discrete and non-intrusive, thereby providing convenience and easy access.
- Promotion: Used to recruit mothers for the program. Public relations using publicity and media releases were used, as well as direct communication on online forums.

8. Audience segmentation: MumBubConnect appealed to mothers in the medium (four days to eight weeks) and long (eight weeks to six months) postnatal periods. This covers the transition from hospital to community and prior to the return to work for the majority of women.

USING SMS IN BREASTFEEDING

Typically, the tangible support offered for women to support breastfeeding behaviors takes the form of face-to-face advice from health professionals, peer counseling via non-profit organizations, such as the Australian Breastfeeding Association, and provision of information through websites, pamphlets, and books. Prior research indicates that face-to-face support is more effective than telephone contact (Britton, McCormic, Renfrew, Wade, & King, 2009; Hall Moran, Edwards, Dykes, & Downe, 2007). Combinations of lay and professional support have also been found to be more effective in improving breastfeeding behaviors than either type of support on its own (Britton et al., 2009). It would appear that very little research has investigated the use of other service delivery channels, such as online discussion forums and m-technologies, in improving breastfeeding behaviors. Given the increasing costs associated with the provision of personalized face-to-face professional support and the need for some women to maximize privacy, discretion, and judgment-free consultations, there is a gap that could be filled by the use of m-technologies, such as text messaging and other social media.

Text messaging (SMS) using mobile phones has been used effectively in health for behaviors such as increasing adherence to treatment programs and is being increasingly used in preventative health (Fjeldsoe, Marshall, & Miller, 2009). For preventative health, SMS has been used in promoting safe sex (Levine, 2007), physical activity (Hurling et al., 2007), smoking cessation (Holman, 2009; Obermayer, Riley Asif, & Jersino, 2004), and diet (Shapiro et al., 2008; Tanguay & Heywood, 2007). Use of mobile phones as a service delivery channel is one of the few technological options with high coverage and pervasiveness across socioeconomic, age, and gender, therefore making it a viable option for broad public health programs (Holman, 2009; Tanguay & Heywood, 2007). Specifically, text messaging offers the benefits of immediacy, privacy, accessibility, convenience, and personalization (Fogg & Eckles, 2007). To date, text messaging has not been used in the context of influencing breastfeeding behaviors, predominantly due to the perceived need for face-to-face contact and the reduced effectiveness of telephone contact. We propose that m-technology for improving breastfeeding behaviors is effective, as it combines the personalized aspects of face-to-face contact, but maintains levels of privacy, is immediate, portable, and overcomes barriers associated with embarrassment. In addition, text messaging is outbound and interactive rather than relying on consumer-initiated calls, which require a high level of self-efficacy and an admittance of failure. There is evidence that when women feel disempowered and helpless in managing breastfeeding they stop, and when women feel confident, they breastfeed longer (Dennis & Faux, 1999; Ertem, Votto, & Leventhal, 2001; Nichols, Schutte, Brown, Dennis, & Price, 2009). The use of text messaging in this study aimed to facilitate the seeking of social support using m-technology to assist women's coping during breastfeeding challenges. Text messages can potentially increase self-efficacy through messages that normalize breastfeeding problems. The automation feature of SMS can remove perceived judgment and thus reduce embarrassment.

Developing the MumBubConnect Social Marketing Program

In partnership with the ABA and a creative director, who came with expertise in digital media, the research team used focus group data to develop a branded, two-way SMS text messaging service, with a website for registration and information accompanied by a supporting social networking site. There were five steps in implementing this program:

1. Gaining consumer insight—focus groups.

2. Developing the brand, SMS system, web, and social networking sites.

3. Recruiting mothers.

4. Piloting.

5. Evaluating.

Gaining Consumer Insight

Focus groups and surveys were used to provide formative and evaluative data of the MumBubConnect concept. Five focus groups were conducted in November and December 2009, with 29 women who had fed an infant with either breastmilk or formula. The purpose of the focus groups was to identify the particular challenges facing women in feeding their infants, potential implementation issues that may prevent successful use of m-technologies, and to refine the content of the messages and key words. In-depth results of these focus groups are reported elsewhere (Gallegos, Russell-Bennett, & Previte, 2011). For the purposes of MumBubConnect, development, mobile phone experiences, attitudes towards social marketing SMS campaigns, and opinions of the messages are summarized in Figures 14.2, 14.3, and 14.4.

Figure 14.2. Mobile Phone Experiences

Mobile Phone Experiences

- Younger mothers
    - Use the mobile phone as an essential link with their peers, family, and friends and did not set any limits on when the phone could be used or how.
    - These women thought text messages would be an ideal way to send and receive messages about breastfeeding.
- Older mothers
    - Do not tend to use mobile phones as their main form of interaction, but rather reserved it for emergencies.
    - These women did not necessarily want to receive text messages at any time of day and stated they would prefer not to be contacted immediately after birth.
    - This group preferred to have a personalized message and not a generic text.
    - They did not tend to send a lot of text messages and most disliked text language.

Figure 14.3. Attitudes Toward Social Marketing SMS Campaigns

Attitudes Towards Social Marketing SMS Campaigns

- Overall the response to a social marketing campaign using text messaging was positive.
- Women were receptive to receiving text messages about breastfeeding, especially if this was linked to a resource where they could access further information.
- The older women liked the idea of a website, which meant they could control access.
- Text messages should be sent in the morning, not during the late afternoon or evening
- There should be no expectation of an immediate response.

Figure 14.4. Opinions of the Messages

Opinions of the Messages

- Each of the messages and key words were initially developed with input from nutrition, breastfeeding, and social marketing experts, as well as the creative director.
- These messages and key words were tested with the women who were positive about the responses to difficulties and the strategies to manage these, but suggested the following changes:
  - o Language was reworked to remove anything that was considered patronizing.
  - o Two phone numbers were given for further support – one was the ABA and the other a Women's Health line aimed to provide non-partisan assistance.
  - o Changes were made to the name of the program to reflect a more personal and less mechanistic approach, thus the proposed brand of Mumsconnex was further developed into MumBubConnect, and a full branding strategy and logo was developed with a creative director.

Developing the Brand, SMS System, Web, and Social Networking Sites

A brief was developed with the creative director that had the strategic objective of being mother-oriented, personalized, digital, providing positive support, and limiting guilt. The brief was to develop a concept that utilized a digital intervention to:

- Trial the impact of a breastfeeding support program provided via m-technology that positively impacted on emotions felt and levels of self-confidence towards breastfeeding.

- Increase the level of women who breastfed their baby with any amount of breastmilk.

- Build in evaluation mechanisms to assess the outputs, outcomes, and impact of the SMS-based support.

The brand "MumBubConnect" with logo was developed (see Figure 14.5). The MBC acronym was accompanied by the positioning statement of "Making Better Connections." This was devised to clearly communicate a key priority of the MumBubConnect initiative and worked as a dual reference to connections between mother and baby and connections between mother and social/health support services. The text messages and responses were tailored and tested using focus groups.

Figure 14.5. MumBubConnect logo

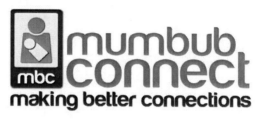

The two-way SMS support system used a "keyword" based "recognition and response" algorithm. The keywords and the responses were developed by the Australian Breastfeeding Association and refined by the research team and creative director. In response to a text from the MBC system inquiring how breastfeeding was going, mothers replied by texting a keyword (one of 20) to indicate how they were managing. The system replied immediately with a response, providing tips, advice, positive reinforcement, and access to help-lines. If women indicated they were experiencing difficulties that may have indicated an underlying mental health issue or significant breastfeeding challenges, the ABA help-line was then notified and an outbound counseling phone call was made. This is the first time outbound calls were used by the ABA to initiate problem solving. The system incorporated built in mechanisms to provide reporting and assessment of a participant's behavior in "real-time."

Recruiting Participants

Women were recruited via a media campaign (print media and radio) and through snowballing, and were required to register on the website, www.mumbubconnect.com.au (Figure 14.6). Women signed up for the service after completion of a baseline survey. Ideally, recruitment for the program could be through antenatal programs and immediately post birth via maternity hospitals and other health professionals. This option, however, was not available for the initial trial.

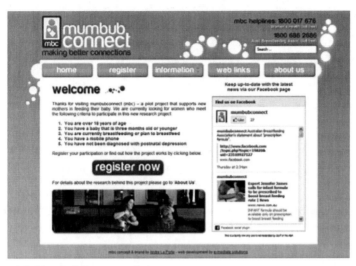

Figure 14.6. MumBubConnect website

Piloting the Program

The mothers received weekly text messages delivered over an eight-week period requiring them to indicate how their breastfeeding was progressing. The women were then required to text back a keyword from a set of responses on a card. At the completion of the eight weeks, women were asked to complete another survey and received a small gift for their infants.

Evaluating the Program

In order to identify any changes in social support seeking behavior and self-efficacy and to obtain attitudes towards the use of text messaging in breastfeeding, a repeated measures approach was adopted with pre- and post-surveys administered. Of the 130 women who registered and completed the pre-survey, six withdrew before commencement and four ceased participation after commencement, with all remaining women (120) completing the post-survey, achieving a 95% response rate.

DEMOGRAPHICS

The mean age of the sample was 31.2 years, which is representative of the population, as the mean age of women giving birth in Australia is 30.7 years (Australian Bureau of Statistics, 2007b). The mean age of infants was 6.7 weeks, which is about the time when women return to work and when breastfeeding rates start to decline (Australian Health Ministers' Conference, 2009; Australian Institute of Family Studies, 2008). This sample, therefore, is the precise group of women that social marketing programs need to target if breastfeeding cessation is to be decreased. Almost all the women were in a relationship with the father of the baby (95%), and the majority of women (92%) were born in Australia. This sample was a relatively well-educated group, with 60% having attended university (compared with nearly 23% of the Australian population generally) (Australian Bureau of Statistics, 2009) and had above average household incomes compared to the Australian median of $1,027 per household per week (Australian Bureau of Statistics, 2007a). Breastfeeding is not a behavior that can be easily recommenced once ceased, thus to be included in the project, all women needed to be offering their baby some breastmilk at the start of the project. Of these women, 83% were fully breastfeeding.

FEEDING BEHAVIOR

Based on a 24-hour recall, at the end of the eight-week period (where the majority of babies were approximately three months old), 93% of women were still feeding their infants some breastmilk (either fully or partially), and 79% of babies were being fully breastfed eight weeks later (a decrease of 4%). This level of fully-breastfed babies is well above the national level of 46% for three-month-old infants (Australian Institute of Family Studies, 2008). Table 14.1 illustrates the changes in other measures.

Table 14.1. Changes in Breastfeeding Measures

Measure	Pre-intervention	Post-intervention	Significance
Self-efficacy	4.00 (score)	4.15 (score)	t= 2.89, p<0.01
Social support seeking behavior	4.02 (score)	4.18 (score)	t= 3.68, p<0.01
Attitudinal loyalty	25 %	32%	X^2= 53.12, p<0.000
Behavioral loyalty	90.9%	92.4%	p=0.5 (ns)
Positive emotions	4.23	4.35	t=2.23, p<0.05
Negative emotions (feeling challenged)	2.47	2.08	t=3.18, p< 0.001

BEHAVIORAL AND PSYCHOLOGICAL MEASURES

Behavioral and psychological measures involved social support seeking behavior (Vitaliano et al., 1985), self-efficacy (Dennis & Faux, 1999), attitudinal and behavioral breastfeeding loyalty (Parkinson, Russell-Bennett, & Previte, 2010), and emotions experienced—hope, joy, anxiety, guilt, challenge (Passyn & Sujan, 2006). Measures of process and impact evaluation were included.

Process Evaluation

Women in the study stated that the keywords were easy to remember. They felt in control when responding to the messages and would have liked them to have been more frequent and to have continued for a longer period of time. They indicated their preference for sending messages at any time without having to wait for a prompt. The mean scores for two impact items—*"the SMS encouraged me to continue breastfeeding"* and *"the messages made me feel more in control"* were five out of a possible seven. The program also prompted half of the women to contact the Australian Breastfeeding Association to seek advice, and of these women, 77% indicated they continued breastfeeding as a result of the contact. Five percent of women received an outbound call. All the women indicated that they used the web to find health information and information about babies, with 84% using the web for health information at least once a week. The overall cost to the women for the program relating to SMS was less than $2.50(AUD) based on maximum SMS charges for the eight-week period.

The qualitative comments about the program were overwhelmingly positive: *"I felt reassured when my bub was feeding constantly, as my response gave me information that told me things were normal";* and *"made me feel as though I was a part of a group. Being isolated in the country I had no mothers group, so enjoyed being acknowledged."*

Lessons Learned

The primary lesson from this research is that SMS is a viable modality for providing point of behavior support and improving self-efficacy that maintains breastfeeding behaviors. In addition:

- SMS is considered to be low tech due to the ubiquitous nature of a range of technologies; however, SMS has broad application as:
  ◊ It is accessible regardless of phone type.
  ◊ It is more accessible in regional and remote areas and has potential in developing countries as well.
  ◊ It is useable across all levels of disadvantage with minimum costs.
- There is a need to upgrade from key words to free text to enhance applicability.
- There are opportunities for value adding with a range of features, including downloadable video, images, and other applications.

- This type of service still needs to be used in conjunction with other strategies that ensure protection, promotion, and monitoring of breastfeeding.

CONCLUSION

This program demonstrated that text messaging is an effective social marketing tool that influences two key determinants of breastfeeding: social support-seeking behaviors and self-efficacy. Australian mothers in this study were very receptive to m-technology and were extremely positive towards the use of text messaging as a breastfeeding support service.

The MumBubConnect program reduced the "social price" of breastfeeding to mothers by increasing self-confidence through offering access to a social support network that was private and reduced embarrassment and guilt. This campaign effectively enabled women to develop personal mastery through the use of verbal persuasion and assurance that they could achieve a good outcome (Bandura, 1977).

Conventional peer support offered by government for breastfeeding mothers typically relies on face-to-face encounters, which is highly labor-intensive and costly (Britton et al., 2009). Often, this type of service is limited to first-time mothers or to postpartum mothers for a limited time. As a way of reducing the cost constraints of support, peer support is often provided by volunteer organizations (for example, the Australian Breastfeeding Association); however, these groups with their specific breastfeeding focus can alienate women who are struggling and, therefore, tend not to be widely used by the broader population. With the ubiquitous spread of the Internet and mobile devices across all demographics (World Bank, 2009), the opportunity to offer innovative, technology-enabled, professional/peer-support for breastfeeding offers substantial value for mothers.

This program demonstrates that m-technology in the form of text messaging has the potential to provide real-time social support and strategies for improving self-efficacy for mothers, regardless of their education, socioeconomic status, or geographical location, given the wide-spread use of mobile phones.

ACKNOWLEDGEMENTS

This research was funded by the Queensland Government Gambling Community Benefit Fund. We would like to acknowledge the project team and the extensive involvement of Ms. Robyn Hamilton, Director, Australian

194 The 10th Step and Beyond: Mother Support for Breastfeeding

Breastfeeding Association, and Mr. André La Porte, from André La Porte Creative Communications. We would also like to thank Joy Parkinson for research assistance and maintaining the MumBubConnect Facebook page, and Ryan McAndrew for research assistance.

Chapter Fifteen

Identifying and Overcoming Barriers to the 10th Step in Lalitpur, India

Komal P. Kushwaha, MD, FIAP
Professor & Head, Department of Pediatrics
BRD Medical College
Gorakhpur, India

Breastfeeding is the most important child survival strategy. Yet exclusivity of breastfeeding during the first six months is not common. The majority of mothers do not breastfeed exclusively because they do not learn the skills of breastfeeding. The Baby-Friendly Hospital Initiative (BFHI) addresses the need for implanting breastfeeding culture in the maternity facility through training of health workers and adopting "The Ten Steps to Successful Breastfeeding." The 10th Step, "Foster the establishment of breastfeeding support groups and refer mothers to them on discharge from the hospital or clinic," has remained the step receiving the least attention, mostly without an integrated program. Integration of Baby-Friendly health facilities with community-based Mother Breastfeeding Support Groups is essential for improving infant and young child feeding status.

INTRODUCTION

Breastfeeding intervention is a most effective strategy for child health, nutrition, and survival. The International Code of Marketing of Breastmilk Substitutes (WHO, 1981) puts responsibility of giving correct and consistent information to pregnant women and mothers on Governments (Article 4.1). Breastfeeding's health benefits and the emotional satisfaction to mothers are also important (Innocenti Declaration, 1990). The Innocenti Declaration on the protection, promotion, and support of breastfeeding sets a global goal for governments for a minimum intervention. The "Ten Steps to Successful Breastfeeding" (WHO/UNICEF, 1989) were endorsed in the Innocenti Declaration and became the foundation of Baby-Friendly Hospital Initiative (BFHI) (WHO/UNICEF, 1991, 2009). The 10th Step is, "Foster the establishment of breastfeeding support groups and refer mothers to them on discharge from the hospital or clinic." This step is needed to ensure ongoing assessment of feeding, identification of difficulties, support for breastfeeding, and maintaining breastfeeding mothers' confidence in the community. The leaders of such mother support groups need to be trained, experienced in breastfeeding, and supervised regularly by institutional experts. They should have access to a BFHI health/maternity facility that provides help to breastfeeding mothers, in order to get reoriented regularly and to have the opportunity to support new mothers in the facility.

New Commitments

During the anniversary of the Innocenti Declaration in 2005 in Florence, Italy, the commitment to breastfeeding and other aspects of Infant and Young Child Feeding were renewed. It was further emphasized that support should be provided for exclusive breastfeeding for six months and continued breastfeeding up to two years of age or beyond in all sectors and at every place. The *Global Strategy for Infant and Young Child Feeding* (WHO/UNICEF, 2003) encourages a "full scale program" to support breastfeeding and other aspects of Infant and Young Child Feeding (IYCF) in all sectors and all places. It highlights the importance of regular community-based programs to provide community and home-based individual counseling and support through well-trained community counselors—the "Mother Support."

Mother Support

In a program to support IYCF, breastfeeding support is a very sensitive issue that requires (i) very special communication skills; (ii) building and sustaining mothers' confidence; (iii) involving family members in this effort; (iv) assessing a breastfeed and other feeding situations by observing feeding, taking the feeding history and weighing the baby; and (v) thereafter providing help to mothers as necessary. Mothers need answers to their individual worries and solutions to feeding difficulties and breast conditions. They may also need to learn positioning of the baby for good attachment at breast, expression of breastmilk, *katori* feeding of milk, tube feeding, preparation of any replacement feed, and preparation of complementary feed and feeding technique. (A *katori* is a small, spouted cup.) Traditional support by elderly women in the family and community is not easily available in many countries, and the women usually lack scientific information and skill.

Mother support groups in the community may include traditional birth attendants, experienced mothers, and community health/nutrition workers. Three to four such members may create a "mother support group" for a population of 500–1000. They should be trained in the basic skills of communication and infant and young child feeding, with training specially developed for them. Such community groups need support and reorientation by another group of counselors-cum-trainers based at a basic health and medical health facility unit. They are designated "facility level counselors" and "trainers" of mother support groups. Facility level trainers require in-depth training in the skill of counseling about infant and young child feeding by experts and experienced trainers for IYCF counseling from medical, nursing, and nutrition backgrounds. The mother support should be available 24 hours a day throughout the year, and they should preferably have a place or office where breastfeeding mothers may seek help. Peer support groups operated by trained mothers, mother support groups operated by women in collaboration with health/nutrition professionals, and mother-to-mother support groups' operated by mothers are three different forms of mother support.

EVIDENCE

While there is a need for published data evaluating the effect of mother support groups embodied in a program, there is good evidence to show that counseling mothers during pregnancy and postnatally, both by health workers and trained lay mother support groups, is effective in increasing breastfeeding indicators. Support for breastfeeding mothers has been vastly reviewed recently. Britton and colleagues (2007) analyzed 34 research reports from 14 countries involving 29,385 mothers receiving breastfeeding support for variable periods, which showed a positive impact on exclusive breastfeeding (in particular) and any breastfeeding rates. A combination of community-level mother support (lay support) and professional support is more effective than professional support alone. One-to-one support is more effective than telephonic support (Britton, McCormick, Renfrew, Wade, & King, 2007; Dykes, 2005).

A systemic review in which the search was limited to articles published in Finnish, Swedish, and English in the 2000–2006 period examined breastfeeding support interventions (Hannula, Kaunonen, & Tarkka, 2008). Interventions that covered the period from pregnancy through to the postnatal period were more effective than interventions of short duration. The effective interventions in pregnancy were interactive ones, such as conversation. Home visits, telephone support, and breastfeeding centers combined with peer support were found to be the most effective. A non-randomized study in KwaZulu-Natal, South Africa, also used home visits by lay counselors from pregnancy through age six months to improve rates of exclusive breastfeeding at four months, in both HIV-infected and uninfected women (Bland et al., 2008).

To evaluate the effect of community-based peer counselors on exclusive breastfeeding, a randomized trial was done in Dhaka, Bangladesh (Haider, Ashworth, Kabir, & Huttly, 2000). Intervention was community-based counseling by peer counselors, who were local mothers given 40 hours training based on the WHO/UNICEF breastfeeding counseling-training course (WHO, 1993) and the book, *Helping Mothers to Breastfeed* (King, 1992). This intervention involved 15 counseling visits to mothers' homes by peer counselors until infants reached five months, starting with two visits in the last trimester of pregnancy, and three in the first two weeks of life (Haider et al., 2000). The prevalence of exclusive breastfeeding at five months was 70 % for the intervention group and 6 % for the control group (p>0.0001). The mothers who received peer counseling initiated breastfeeding earlier than the other mothers, with lower use of pre-lacteal foods (Haider et al., 2000).

A study by Bhandari and colleagues in India (2003) assessed the feasibility, effectiveness, and safety of an educational intervention to promote exclusive breastfeeding. The study group developed the intervention through formative research, pair-matching eight communities on their baseline characteristics. One of each pair was randomized to receive the intervention, the other acting as a control. Training in counseling was given to health and nutrition workers in the intervention communities to support exclusive breastfeeding. The training module used and counseling schedule were not specified.

At three months, exclusive breastfeeding rates were 79% in the intervention group and 48% in the control group (p< 0.0001). A lower seven-day diarrhea prevalence was recorded in the intervention communities, compared with the control communities at three months (p=0.028) and six months (p=0.04). The mean measures of growth at age three months and six months were similar between groups (Bhandari et al., 2003).

A study evaluating the effect of postnatal peer counseling on exclusive breastfeeding of low birth weight infants was done in the Philippines in 2004 (Agrasada, 2005). Two hundred and four mothers were randomized into three groups—two intervention groups receiving home-based counseling visits and a control group of mothers who did not receive counseling. One intervention group received visits by counselors trained in breastfeeding counseling (WHO training course) and the other by counselors trained in general childcare. At six months, 44% of the mothers given breastfeeding counseling, 7% of childcare counseled mothers, and no mothers in the control group were exclusively breastfeeding. Mothers in the breastfeeding counseling group were more likely than other mothers to still be breastfeeding at six months.

Other studies have measured the positive effects of interventions on a broader scale on two continents, Africa and Latin America (Quinn, 2005), or described local programs (Semega-Janneh, 2005).

Unfortunately, peer-counseling visits from outsiders in HIV settings may lead to fear and suspicion of the workers' intentions, according to a qualitative study in South Africa of how women in three communities experienced an infant-feeding peer counseling intervention (Nor et al., 2009). Yet, other women in the study, especially those with HIV, valued the emotional support provided by peer counseling.

These studies highlight the importance of good practical skill training, counseling, the presence of local women in the support group, skilled supervision, a supportive health system and administration, the presence of referral centers and timely referral, frequent post-natal contacts (eight to nine), regular orientation, refresher courses, and incentives for the work.

THE LALITPUR PROJECT

A novel model of mother support groups based in the community and structured in the health and nutrition delivery system has been introduced in the District of Lalitpur, Uttar Pradesh, India. This has been described in a report by the present author:

> This is an ongoing project in District Lalitpur, reaching out to children under two years in a population of one million, with more than 30,000 annual births. The project is establishing a system of universal reach with infant feeding counseling, improved supervision, convergence, and resultant change in feeding behaviors.

> [The area has] a very high infant mortality and high levels of under-nutrition in children, very low rates of optimal breastfeeding practices, and poor healthcare indicators for children. The intervention utilized community-based as well as facility-based strategies for promotion of optimal IYCF

practices through skilled counseling, better supervision, and monitoring with the aim of reaching out to all pregnant and lactating women to contribute to the nutrition and health status of their children under two (Kashwaha, 2010).

The infant feeding counseling was provided at family level, with a support system at block and district level. Forty-eight local graduate men and women "mentors" were trained as trainers, using a seven-day training course, *The "3 in 1" training program: Capacity building initiative for building health workers' skills in infant and young child feeding counseling training course* (BPNI/IBFAN, 2009). This course, developed by the Breastfeeding Promotion Network of India (BPNI) and the International Baby Food Action Network (IBFAN), covered breastfeeding counseling, complementary feeding counseling, and HIV and infant feeding counseling. These mentors provided support at block and district level counseling centers (Figures 15.1 and 15.2). They each trained a team of three to four village level counselors from among Anganwadi workers, ASHA (Accredited Social Health Activist), Dai (Traditional Birth Attendants), or a link mother from the same village, who formed a "Mother Support Group" (MSG). They did home visiting and facility-based counseling to provide education to mothers and families on breastfeeding and complementary feeding (Figure 15.3). The village level counselors helped and supported mothers with feeding difficulties, and referred them to block level counseling centers if they were not able to solve any problems (Kashwaha, 2010, p. 1). The pre-intervention (2006) and post intervention (2009) evaluation showed significant improvement in four feeding practices; namely, reduction in pre-lacteal feeding (from 44.4% to 15%), increase in initiation of breastfeeding within one hour of birth (from 39.2% to 72%), exclusive breastfeeding for the first six months (from 6.85% to 50%), and introduction of complementary foods along with continued breastfeeding between six to nine months (from 4.6% to 85%).

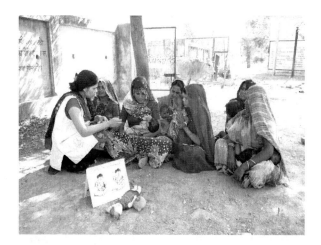

Figure 15.1. Small group, Lalitpur project.

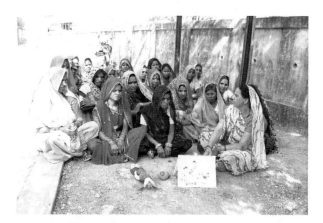

Figure 15.2. Training, Lalitpur project.

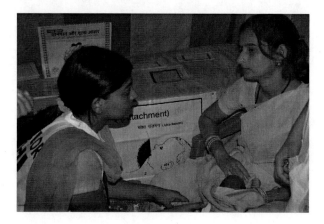

Figure 15.3. One-on-one support, Lalitpur project.

The mentors and village level counselors were found to be supportive and enjoyed good rapport within the community. The project reach was nearly universal, as 84-90 percent of mothers reported having received advice on various infant feeding practices by AWWs (63-67%), ASHAs (16-21%), and Dais (5-16%). Thus the project has created a favorable atmosphere for continuation of such activities, with the provision of counseling firmly in place (Kashwaha, 2010, p. 3). It has demonstrated a real convergence at village level and heightened motivation of workers to prevent malnutrition and the morbidity associated with it in infants and young children. This project has also revealed that women can be identified and trained locally, so they can do home visits with some incentives. Establishing a system of nearly universal reach is possible in the existing health and nutrition delivery system through additional human resources and good quality training and supervision.

The Mother Support "10th Step" of BFHI is crucial to any health and nutrition program. The recommendations are in place. There is plenty of evidence in its support, but emphasis is poor and direction is missing. The Lalitpur model is a novel approach in this direction, highlighting the need for additional manpower and budgetary allocation.

Conclusion

Breastfeeding is the most important child survival strategy. Yet exclusivity of breastfeeding during the first six months is not common. The majority of mothers do not breastfeed exclusively because they do not learn the skills of breastfeeding. The Baby-Friendly Hospital Initiative (BFHI) addresses the need for implanting breastfeeding culture in the maternity facility through training of health workers and adopting "The Ten Steps to Successful Breastfeeding." The 10th Step, "Foster the establishment of breastfeeding support groups and refer mothers to them on discharge from the hospital or clinic," has remained the step receiving the least attention, mostly without an integrated program. Integration of Baby-Friendly health facilities with community-based Mother Breastfeeding Support Groups is essential for improving infant and young child feeding status.

Acknowledgement

The manuscript has been prepared with help from Dr. Priyanka Jaiswal, Lecturer, BRD Medical College, Gorakhpur, UP, India and Mr. Praveen Dubey, the Personal Assistant.

Chapter Sixteen

Breastfeeding Peer Counselors in South Africa: Influences of Local Factors

Jean Ridler, RN, RM, IBCLC
Rosemary Gauld, RN, RM, IBCLC, ICCE

INTRODUCTION

South Africa is known as the Rainbow Nation due to the cultural, ethnic, creed, and language diversity of the population. The country has eleven official languages, making health information delivery a challenge. Cape Town is the legislative capital of the South Africa and is the capital of the Western Cape, a province to the southwest of the country. With its famous landmarks of Table Mountain and Cape Point, it is a very popular destination for tourists. As of 2011 (Wikipedia, 2011), the city had an estimated population of 5.8 million.

The five underlying natural causes of death common for infants and children are: intestinal infectious diseases, influenza and pneumonia, malnutrition, other acute lower respiratory infections, and certain disorders involving the immune mechanism (Statistics South Africa, 2010).

The healthcare system consists of both a public and a private sector to meet the needs of the population. The Western Cape Department of Health delivers a comprehensive package of health services to the people of the province. The Primary Healthcare Services consist of 479 facilities in 32 sub-districts and six districts. The hospital services include 34 district, eight regional, and three tertiary hospitals. Some of the categories of those entitled to free medical services include: children under the age of six, pregnant women, children who have been placed in care, and unemployed people.

Midwife Obstetric Units

Groote Schuur hospital is a large, government-funded teaching hospital situated on the slopes of Devil's Peak in Cape Town. Famous for being the institution where Dr. Christiaan Barnard conducted the first human heart transplant, it is affiliated with the University of Cape Town. It is the tertiary referral center for the Southern Cape Peninsula. The mothers present with a large range of obstetric and medical problems, and the incidence of preterm birth is high. Skin-to-skin care of these infants and provision of mother's own milk is highly encouraged. A lodger ward is available where mothers can stay. Sadly, due to the distance from home, cost of travel, and the need to return to paid employment, many mothers do not stay with their babies and prefer to take their maternity leave once the baby is discharged from hospital. Support in the community to continue expressing milk is vital. Babies are usually referred to their local Midwife Obstetric Units (MOUs) for follow-up care upon discharge from Groote Schuur hospital and are also given contact details of a peer counselor (PC).

The urgent need for an alternative to domiciliary delivery in Cape Town has been met by the development of MOUs. These primary care units are situated in suburbs with a high population density. They are staffed entirely by midwives and are linked by telephone to the base hospital. A flying squad service is available at the regional center (e.g., the maternity block at Groote Schuur Hospital). Regular visits are made to the units by the medical staff. Strict criteria for delivery at the MOUs have resulted in a very low perinatal mortality rate, and the units have at the same time relieved the serious overcrowding in the teaching hospitals. The concept of the MOU is particularly suited to Africa and, indeed, to any developing country.

Women giving birth at the MOUs are discharged after six hours, which makes the role of the PC vitally important. Good antenatal breastfeeding education given by the PCs, while women are waiting to see the midwife, ensures that new mothers are better prepared when they return home with their new babies. The support the PCs give to these mothers within the community is invaluable.

The Peer Counselor Training Program in Cape Town: Beginnings

St Monica's was a small maternity hospital situated in the heart of Cape Town on the slopes of Table Mountain until its closure in 2000. In 1992 the hospital began working towards Baby-Friendly status, the first hospital in South Africa to take this step. This hospital catered to mothers from a wide geographical area and, therefore, in order to fulfill Step 10, they identified mothers from these areas suitable for training. Consequently, La Leche League ran the first Peer Counseling Program (PCP) in Cape Town in 1993. It was probably the first hospital to admit mothers of preterm infants (born elsewhere) to a "kangaroo ward" to help establish breastfeeding. St Monica's became South Africa's first Baby-Friendly Hospital in 1994, with their plaque being presented by James P. Grant of UNICEF.

In March 1994, the PCP was rolled out in earnest at St Monica's, and this yielded 148 PCs. These numbers steadily increased as the demand for the PCP developed to fill the need for breastfeeding support for the mothers. Mothers were referred to PCs in their communities, who were likely to speak the same language and understand cultural beliefs and values.

MALE PEER COUNSELORS

One of the female PCs who trained very early in the program carried out home visits in her community. As these visits were sometimes late at night, her husband, Arnold, accompanied her. While she was helping the mother, Arnold would chat with the baby's father about the wonders of breastfeeding. He realized that with more information he could become a valuable resource and provide advice that was consistent with what the female PCs were providing. He was thus invited to train as a PC. Arnold did not actively help women, but could counsel over the phone if his wife was not available and was a wonderful breastfeeding advocate in the community he served. Shortly after this, a young male nutrition advisor attended a PC course and proved to be an enthusiastic breastfeeding advocate and educator. Another young male PC was well accepted in a poor farming community and actively helped mothers to breastfeed. In this particular community, bare breasts are not sexualized and women are not embarrassed at having a male PC.

Next came the training of over 100 Community Health Workers (CHWs) from Khayelitsha, a large township of over one million mainly Xhosa-speaking inhabitants outside Cape Town. These CHWs were identified and recommended by their communities. They received some basic primary healthcare education and a small stipend from the Department of Health (DoH). Their main functions were tuberculosis treatment compliance and visiting mothers with newborns. A community-based neonatologist recognized that breastfeeding education was needed and several PC courses were run over the next few years.

Many of these community health workers were male. In this community, too, breasts are not considered as sexual objects and upper body nudity is not frowned upon. Role playing during the course was very real—with male PCs assisting female participants to "attach" a doll to the bare breast. The La Leche League International Peer Counselor Program was adapted in 1996 to a new course based on the Wellstart Training Curriculum for community-based breastfeeding support, as these teaching methods were more suited to the training of the Community Health Workers. The course was very interactive and drew strongly on the knowledge and wisdom of the health workers regarding the child health problems experienced within their communities and the connection of these problems to lack of breastfeeding.

It is within the cultural context that solutions that underline infant feeding problems must ultimately emerge. Changes, if they are to last, need to originate from within a culture, not be imposed from without. These Community Health Workers learned well from storytelling and role playing, and imparted important messages to their community via beautifully harmonized songs. The male PCs worked mainly in Khayelitsha, assisting women who gave birth in the MOUs, Groote Schuur hospital, or St Monica's hospital. Some of the male PCs attended the La Leche League National Conferences where they shared their passion via poems and songs.

Exclusive Breastfeeding

Breastfeeding is traditional in the Khayelitsha community. It is seen as both nurturing and functional, with many babies being breastfed for three to four years. However, *exclusive* breastfeeding was extremely rare, hence the prevalence of diarrhea and pneumonia. The main focus of the PCP in this area was on exclusive breastfeeding for six months, and the PCs had a profound effect, with exclusive breastfeeding becoming almost the norm in this community. The PCP rapidly expanded to communities served by other MOUs. In these areas the PCs were mainly female.

Funding

A generous grant from one of the oil companies sustained the running of the PCP. Due to good record keeping and accountability, this grant was renewed. Training materials and transport costs were covered and La Leche League Leaders gave of their time freely.

The Focus Changes

With the advent of HIV/AIDS and its high prevalence in the Khayelitsha and other high-density areas, most of the Community Health Workers were sent for training in this. Funding for HIV/AIDS programs was readily available from local and international sponsors. HIV/AIDS counselors could therefore receive an adequate salary instead of the previous small stipend. In spite of the local and national Prevention of Mother to Child Transmission (PMtCT) policies stating that the infant feeding choice should be that of the mother, the HIV/AIDS counselors were led to believe that breastmilk should not be given to babies born to HIV positive mothers, with the focus being on transmission rates rather than health outcomes. If mothers did not breastfeed, replacement feeding had to be Acceptable, Feasible, Affordable, Sustainable and Safe, for which the acronym AFASS was used. These conditions could mostly not be met in the informal areas of Khayelitsha, as is the case in other areas of the country (Coutsoudis, Coovadia, & Wilfert, 2009). The term AFASS has now been replaced in line with the latest WHO recommendations on infant feeding in the context of HIV and AIDS. The following seven identified criteria must be met for safe formula feeding:

1. The mother is clinically well.

2. Safe water and sanitation are assured at the household level and in the community.

3. The mother, or caregiver, can reliably provide sufficient formula milk to support normal growth and development of the baby.

4. The mother, or caregiver, can prepare the formula hygienically and frequently enough so that it is safe and caries a low risk of diarrhea and malnutrition.

5. The mother or caregiver can, in the first six months, exclusively give formula milk.

6. The family is supportive of this practice.

7. The mother or caregiver can access healthcare that offers comprehensive child health services (Yezingane Network & UNICEF, 2011).

As part of the PMtCT program, free infant formula was supplied for the first six months of life by the government, and this had a spillover effect into the community as a whole, resulting in very few mothers exclusively breastfeeding. Of great concern was the large number of women mixed feeding. A large KwaZulu Natal study, including 2722 HIV-infected and non infected women, showed that infants who received both breast and formula milk were twice as likely to become HIV-infected than those infants given breastmilk alone (Coovadia et al., 2007).

Where Are We Now?

The Midwife Obstetric Units in Khayelitsha and other communities are either Baby-Friendly accredited or working towards accreditation. Because of the change in focus, PC numbers are greatly reduced. Currently, the Department of Health funds just 27 PCs to work in these facilities. There are currently no active male peer counselors in breastfeeding programs in the Cape Town area. Most male PCs have been absorbed into the HIV/AIDS arena.

The Future

In the 2010 Millennium Development Goals "Countdown to 2015" Report (WHO/ UNICEF, 2010), South Africa is listed as one of the 12 out of 68 countries not on track to reduce infant mortality. In addition, the country records the lowest exclusive breastfeeding rates in the world.

The National Government has now committed to changing this unacceptable situation. A new strategy that will go a long way to address our appalling statistics is the revised Prevention of Mother-to-Child Transmission guidelines.

National Breastfeeding Consultative Meeting

A National Breastfeeding Consultative Meeting was held August 22-23, 2011, in Pretoria. There were 650 delegates, comprising various stakeholders, academics, researchers, traditional healers, NGO's, health professionals, and others. The Aims and Objectives listed for this meeting were:

- To reposition promotion, protection, and support for breastfeeding as a key child survival strategy in South Africa.

- To build consensus on the direction that the South African Government should take following the WHO recommendations on infant feeding in the context of HIV and AIDS.

- To mobilize support and call for action to improve infant feeding as a key component of child survival.

The focus of the meeting was to be on evidence-based strategies aimed at improving systems at both facility and community level.

Alarming statistics included (Goga et al., 2011):

- At 3 weeks only 20% mothers were exclusively breastfeeding.
- 30% were mixed feeding.
- 15% were exclusively formula feeding.
- The rest were adding cereal to the baby's diet—at three weeks.
- *At six weeks, 80% of HIV positive mothers were mixed feeding.*

At the Consultative Meeting, Dr. Nigel Rollins from the World Health Organization, Geneva, referred to recent studies and stated that policy, interventions, and programs should be judged on their ability to promote HIV-free survival among all children and on the health and survival of mothers. Preventing HIV transmission is not enough. Dr. Tanya Doherty, from the University of Western Cape and the Medical Research Council, calculated that 204 million rand7 will be saved if free formula is withdrawn (except for babies still on the program, who will continue to receive it until they reach six months of age). This will be enough to employ at least 6800 well-trained community counselors.

Clinical Guidelines: Prevention of Mother-to-Child Transmission (National Department of Health, South Africa, 2010) is a well-referenced document that contains clear management guidelines that need to be followed antenatally, during labor and birth, postnatally, at the six-week check-up, and beyond. It also has guidelines on counseling and testing. All HIV-infected pregnant women with a CD4 count of 350 or below will commence lifelong Antiretroviral Therapy. Women who are not eligible for lifelong treatment will start prophylaxis treatment at 14 weeks of pregnancy.

"For the first time, HIV-positive-infected women can safely breastfeed their children, provided the child is taking ARVs during the breastfeeding period," said Dr. Aaron Motsoaledi, Minister of Health. A summary of the proceedings of the Breastfeeding Consultative Meeting can be found in the statement made by the Minister of Health after the meeting (Motsoaledi, 2011). To put things into perspective, Prof. David Saunders shared some facts at the Fifth AIDS Conference:

- 35% of South African under age five deaths are associated with HIV/AIDS.
- This leaves 65 % of deaths due to other conditions.
- Diarrhea and pneumonia are the top two killers of our children.

---

7   The rand is the South African currency.

- These causes of death are much higher in a non-breastfed population.

- An opportunity is now presented to move beyond a focus of preventing HIV transmission to a focus on child survival through vigorously promoting the practice of exclusive breastfeeding.

Dr. Motsoaledi predicted that after the Consultative Meeting, South Africa will never be the same as far as lactating mothers are concerned. Time will tell!

With the new 2010 HIV/AIDS policy (antiretrovirals for both mother and infant) indicating encouragement of exclusive breastfeeding for all babies, perhaps the future will see a change in focus and a return of the male PC.

Chapter Seventeen

Sustainability: Why Good Programs Fail and What We Need to Know

Virginia Thorley, OAM, PhD, IBCLC, FILCA

INTRODUCTION

This chapter will examine conundrums about why some excellent programs fail and what individuals and organizations need to consider in establishing new programs for mother support or evaluating existing ones. Some of the challenges facing groups or programs of any size are: becoming known to mothers who need the support; access to this support, such as where the help is located; inclusiveness, that is, whether the group is welcoming; the financial sustainability of the program; and finding and keeping volunteers who are returning to paid employment. Other programs providing support to very small numbers of mothers whose babies have a relatively unusual challenge may also be difficult to sustain in the community. Indeed, low numbers of babies with a particular condition may make establishing breastfeeding support in the community extremely difficult. All of these factors are important in the sustainability of a group or program, and the lack of any of them can put survival of this support at risk. Yet, it is lack of financial sustainability, especially when a service has been established on short-term funding, which is most likely to lead to failure of good quality programs that are meeting a need.

BECOMING KNOWN

Becoming known is essential for any support group to fulfill its function (Wituk, Ealey, Brown, Shepherd, & Meissen, 2005). Mother support groups and programs need to become known in order to reach the mothers who need breastfeeding support and to continue to provide this support. Often, there is a lack of a clearinghouse to put those who need the service in touch with those who can provide it. Where volunteer hours are involved, the focus is on the support, and consequently, administrative tasks may be a lower priority. So providing contact information to hospitals, well-baby centers, the media, and the public may be sporadic. Contact details posted at health facilities or in the community are sometimes out of date, and the author has seen contact information for volunteers who have moved out of the organization or left the district still on display. Contact information that is old and dusty or consists of a fuzzy photocopy is unattractive and unlikely to be picked up and taken home by the mothers who need the support.

Groups that remain unknown are unable to serve the mothers who need their help and support. Consequently, they are likely to fail, no matter how well the mothers are trained to provide the support. The lesson for breastfeeding support groups is to establish a relationship with maternity facilities, community centers, and other local organizations that can refer mothers to them. Time is also well spent in investigating whether the local newspapers or radio stations offer free community announcements, including meeting times and locations.

ACCESS TO THE SUPPORT

Several questions need to be considered when providing support to mothers in the community, whether this is in cities, smaller towns, or rural areas:

• Is the meeting place easily accessible?

• Is it near public transport or cheap parking?

• Is there access for prams or baby buggies, or for disabled mothers?

• Is the meeting place safe?

Women will be deterred from attending support groups if they find it too hard to attend. The meeting place needs to be easily accessible, perhaps in a location where mothers and babies often go. The Baby Cafés in Britain and elsewhere (see chapter 9) take accessibility very seriously and are located in children's centers, community rooms, and church halls. In Vancouver, Canada, in the early 1990s, women with high-risk pregnancies, poor diets, and low literacy were unable to read public transport timetables to attend a support program, the Friday Lunch Club. So they were provided with assistance in traveling to weekly meetings, where good nutrition and cooking were taught, and local La Leche League mothers provided support on breastfeeding. Today, the Rush Mothers' Milk Club in Chicago (see chapter 12) provides a taxi service to enable mothers of infants in the NICU, especially low-income mothers, to attend the regular Rush Mothers' Milk Club Lunches at which they can find support and information.

Mothers who use prams or baby buggies need ramps to access meeting venues, as steps are a barrier and leaving the pram outside is unacceptable and unsafe. Mothers themselves may have mobility problems and need easy access. Finally, women are reluctant to attend if the meeting place is in a high-crime area, has poor lighting, or is on a busy road that they and their children need to cross.

INCLUSIVENESS

It takes courage for mothers with babies and young children to attend a meeting for the first time, especially if they have no one to go with and everyone at the meeting is a stranger. For some mothers it may be the first time they leave the house with a new baby, a daunting effort for some. The mother may never return if no one greets and welcomes her, or if she feels the other mothers have been unwelcoming or ignored her. An established group with long-term members who have formed a clique may seem unwelcoming to the new would-be member. Yet the women in the clique may wonder why their group fails to attract and keep new members. Groups such as this usually fail when the long-term members move on to other interests. In some situations, mothers may feel more comfortable attending a group where there are women from their own culture or socio-economic group present. Very young mothers can feel out of place in a group where the majority are older mothers.

FINANCIAL SUSTAINABILITY

Mother support groups of all sizes commonly struggle with financial sustainability. Small groups may survive, month by month, on a tiny income—or they may not. If the members are predominantly middle-class, small fundraising strategies among members may work, at least while the core group of mothers is still interested. On the other hand, if groups grow rapidly, their very success creates the need for a larger and more reliable income, and this requires more attention to an administrative structure, which, in turn, requires money to cover expenses. Where the members of the group have low incomes or are otherwise disadvantaged, survival of the group or program will depend on outside funding, perhaps from a hospital or the Department of Health.

Drop-in centers to support breastfeeding mothers may struggle to find ongoing funding. Some are begun as short-term projects and their survival then depends on whether further funding can be found. The Baby Café concept has addressed this challenge by allowing only centers with regular funding to use their brand, and this proviso and the Baby Café "brand" makes the centers attractive to funding bodies (see chapter 9).

Examples abound where self-sustainability has failed when funding of the program has ended or the money has been used to redeploy staff. In Western Cape, South Africa, the breastfeeding PCP provided necessary support to low-income mothers in the townships and rural areas near Cape Town. When the Department of Health's funding priorities changed, the PCs were employed in other programs (see chapter 16). A PCP was established in Townsville in North Queensland to provide breastfeeding support to Australian Aboriginal and Torres Strait Islander mothers. This program met an identified need in the local indigenous community, as indigenous mothers were reluctant to attend other breastfeeding support groups and had a relatively low breastfeeding rate. The funding was not renewed and the program collapsed, despite attempts to find ways to continue it.

Finding New Ways to Generate Income

Large organizations that have continued to survive for many years have learned to change old methods of generating income and develop new ways. For the Australian Breastfeeding Association (ABA, formerly the Nursing Mothers' Association of Australia, or NMAA), finding enough money to cover expenses and provide new services has been a continuing challenge. Membership subscriptions have usually only covered member services, such as the organization's magazine, rather than providing a profit. In the early years when there were very few groups, a modest income was generated in similar ways to those used by other women's organizations of the time. These included sales at meetings of items donated by members, cake stalls in shopping streets, and fashion parades. The development of printed information for breastfeeding mothers soon followed, providing a service and generating a small income. Other products to be added to the sales inventory early in the NMAA's existence were a baby sling, lambskin bedding, and cookbooks. Rapid expansion of the membership in the 1970s, combined with isolation of counselors and members in inland and northern areas, increased the strain on finances. Interest in breastfeeding was rising and more mothers, including non-members, needed the support of the NMAA. Consequently the volunteer counselors were typically carrying a heavy load. Training more counselors, especially in remote and rural areas, was expensive, as some volunteers had to travel long distances to attend workshops and conferences. Money had to be found to make this possible. As an example, for several years members in Cairns, a small city in the tropical north, took on the contract to deliver telephone directories in the local area to raise money to send their breastfeeding counselors to conferences for ongoing training (Thorley, 2009, p. 56). Despite fears of losing control of how the organization functioned, volunteers began to write grant applications, at first to governments at federal, state, and local levels, and then to other funding bodies, such as the gaming industry's community fund.

Since grants, when successful, provided money for a set period or for a specific project or equipment, they could not be relied upon as continuing income. Income from traditional fund-raising methods and sales was too little to fund the association's expansion to meet the increasing needs. New initiatives were needed and included an annual national lottery, appeal letters, and the creation of a trading arm, as a company to sell the association's products and other merchandise.

Two major financial crises impacted on the association and threatened its future (Thorley, 2011b, pp. 197-209). The first was an insurance claim from a minor injury caused by an item rented from the NMAA (now the ABA). After the court case, the association's public liability insurer rejected the claim. An appeal for donations to pay the damages claim was successful in raising the necessary amount of over $[AUD]75,000, from over 4,500 donors (Paterson, 1986, p. 11).

The second financial crisis came when the ABA's budget suffered a loss of $160,000 in the six months to February 2002. So serious was the loss made by the trading subsidiary that the association had to draw on its own money to support it. Strategies used included the hiring of a management consultant and a rigorous cost-cutting exercise, the "100-Day Challenge," which involved members of the association at all levels around the country (Croker, personal communication, March 2012). The loss was gradually clawed back and the 2004-2005 financial year showed a profit for both the association and the trading arm (Australian Breastfeeding Association, 2005). The trading arm's online business and two shops have since been profitable.

Cost-Cutting

Cost-cutting is more than a negative action to curb the loss of money in tight financial times. It can also be part of innovations to reach mothers in different ways, as new technologies become more accessible and affordable. Technology was for many years a barrier in Australia as the cost of long-distance telephone calls and postage was high, and rural or remote areas were late in receiving access to reliable telephone services and the Internet. Now that there is access to email in much of the country, use of electronic communications has reduced some costs. This has benefited the ABA, as breastfeeding counselors and members can now receive messages electronically, saving the association the cost of printing and mailing news and other information. Email counseling has become a very popular way for mothers to reach out for support and information about their breastfeeding challenges or to receive encouragement. While vast distances are a barrier that cannot be completely eliminated, electronic communication has improved the delivery of support to mothers, anyway, while at the same time reducing costs.

OTHER BARRIERS TO SUSTAINABILITY

Finding Enough Volunteers

Mother-to-mother breastfeeding support depends upon a continuing supply of experienced mothers willing to train and volunteer their time to do this work. In countries where expatriates have begun the groups and trained local women, as in Malaysia and Paraguay, they have left the country at the end of their husbands' work contracts (see chapters 6 and 7). In some countries, low incomes and the necessity of contributing to family income has meant that PCS or breastfeeding counselors have been paid a small stipend (see chapters 12 and 16). Otherwise, they are unable to afford to provide time to the program. In groups where the volunteers were in the past mainly middle-class women who were stay-at-home mothers, the pool of volunteers is shrinking, as many women in this demographic have also returned to paid employment (Thorley, 2011b). New strategies explored by the ABA have included having shorter shifts on telephone and email counseling rosters, so that women with full-time employment can continue to provide breastfeeding support. Even so, when numbers of experienced counselors decline, it places a heavy load on fewer women, and that can lead to more resignations.

Different Community Languages

The ability of those supporting the mother to speak the language she best understands is a factor in the effectiveness and acceptability of the support offered. Language differences can be an issue in several situations: firstly, for immigrant mothers, whether they are immigrants from another country or another region of their country where a different language is used; secondly, for mothers in a country where more than one language is used. By way of example, chapter 7 discusses the value of having PCs and other supporters who speak Guarani, the second official language of Paraguay, which is commonly spoken by the less affluent sections of the population. Barriers to mothers' attendance at La Leche League meetings included the fact that the original groups were founded by foreigners, who knew Spanish, but not the second official language. Now some of the Leaders are fluent in Guarani. Other barriers were the reluctance of Paraguayan women to go to a stranger's house for meetings. South Africa, the "rainbow nation," has eleven official languages. One of the values of having breastfeeding PCs when the program was still operating was their ability to support new mothers in the community language (see chapter 16).

Where a Few Babies in the Area Have an Anatomical Challenge

Mothers whose babies have physical challenges that are not common in the community may lack a local breastfeeding support group for their babies' special situation. Mothers of babies with cleft lip and/or palate are an example of this situation. If a small local group forms, the lack of numbers will affect its survival after the founders move on. In New Zealand, a small cleft support group exists in the major city of Auckland and provides information through printed material and a website, but breastfeeding is only a small part of this. Mothers are largely dependent on professional support for issues specific to the particular condition and a regular breastfeeding group for further breastfeeding support. This section draws on my discussion with Bev Pownall and her extensive experience as a hospital-based healthcare professional assisting the mothers of babies with clefts and other oral anomalies.

In New Zealand the 35 or so babies born each year with clefts of the lip and/or palate are spread across the whole country. The largest hospital sees only about 12 such newborns a year. Add to that the fact that their mothers are often deterred from breastfeeding by negative comments from all around them, and it is obvious there is a lack of a pool of experienced mothers who can share their skills and passion for breastfeeding a baby with a cleft.

With antenatal diagnosis of these conditions, preparation before the baby is born is encouraged. Antenatal counseling includes the practicalities of where to hire hospital grade breast pumps. (In New Zealand scheduling the surgery when the infant is several months old is believed to produce better outcomes; therefore, pumping long-term is an option discussed with all mothers). In addition, antenatal counseling provides parents with the opportunity to meet all the professionals who will be helping their babies, and receive information on what sources of support are available in their communities. Writing a plan, in conjunction with the team's IBCLCs (lactation consultants) and the mother's midwife, is encouraged, as mothers can feel overwhelmed after the birth.

The mothers may never have breastfed before, and there is still the belief in the community and among some professionals that breastfeeding or providing expressed breastmilk is out of the question. The Middlemore Hospital in Auckland has Breastfeeding Advocates, mothers from the community who are trained to provide non-professional breastfeeding support and who are remunerated. They are required to be at least bi-lingual. They assist all ethnic groups, but are particularly helpful with Maori and Pacific Islander mothers. They "support, motivate, encourage, explain, provide written information, show [breastfeeding] DVDs, and above all use their own personal experience to relate to women" (Bev Pownall, personal communication, September 2011).

In discharge planning in the hospital, La Leche League and local PC groups are recommended for breastfeeding support, but they have limited experience feeding babies with clefts, as the numbers are small and many mothers do not breastfeed. The hospital lactation consultants discuss with the mothers, antenatally and postnatally, the adaptability of babies and how it may be possible to breastfeed using specific techniques to facilitate negative pressure. They also explain that, if supplementation is needed, it need not be by bottle. Unfortunately, other health professionals still believe that this is impossible and that bottles and teats are essential. Consequently, these negative messages undermine the mother's confidence in her baby's ability to breastfeed. Whom should they believe?

CONCLUSION

This chapter is intended to provide an introduction to some of the issues that make it difficult for groups of any size to survive and to provide real-life examples. I have discussed why good programs sometimes fail and why some groups of mothers are difficult to provide support to, which is specific for their needs. Some groups will survive difficult circumstances, as in one of the examples, by dealing with a crisis and finding ways to improve sustainability.

If a group or program closes while it is still needed, that is a loss for the mothers and babies who could have been helped. My hope is that the ideas presented here lead to discussion among participants in mother support groups and programs. Too many good groups fail because they haven't developed self-sustainability or the ability to reflect and reinvent the group to meet changing needs.

Conclusion

Going Forth From Here

Virginia Thorley, OAM, PhD, IBCLC, FILCA

A concluding chapter can be a rounding off of a discussion, a summary of an argument, an ending. I prefer this conclusion to the book to be a beginning for the reader, not an end. Why so?

The purpose of this book has been to address the issue of providing support to enable mothers to breastfeed their babies. The emphasis has been on encouraging exclusive breastfeeding for about six months and breastfeeding with appropriate, nutrient-dense, locally-available, affordable complementary foods thereafter, for as long as mother and baby wish. Mother support makes it easier for a mother to breastfeed her baby anywhere, anytime, and that may mean overcoming barriers, such as public disapproval and unhelpful industrial conditions. The chapter authors have described a number of barriers to establishing and sustaining effective mother support.

As Melissa Vickers and I, and our support team of Sarah Amin, Rebecca Magalhães, and Paulina Smith, had hoped, our carefully chosen chapter authors have provided information about a broad range of forms that mother support can take. We wanted to start with the 10th Step of the Baby-friendly Hospital Initiative, mother support after she returns home, which in some countries or regions has proven difficult for hospitals to achieve. As the chapters unfolded, we have seen that mother support is not a one-size-fits-all package. It comes in all shapes and forms, and the people who are able to provide that support are just as diverse. When you opened this book, you would have had an idea in your mind, dear reader, of what mother support is, and how your community is—or isn't—providing it. I hope that as you read on, the diverse approaches to breastfeeding support described have opened up more possibilities, some of which may be adaptable in your community or workplace.

Mother-to-mother support is valuable, as is the storytelling and sharing of experiences that is deeply embedded in this form of support; it is an aid to the new mother to breastfeed optimally. We must not forget that the family—an extended family of fathers, grandparents, aunts and uncles, cousins, and siblings—is the original form of mother support. During periods when breastfeeding became rare in some communities, which was the case in many areas during the 20th century, this support was no longer available to many mothers. Indeed, the sort of support provided by the family often undermined breastfeeding because, for several generations, normal infant behavior came to be seen as pathological (the clock ruled). In this climate of belief, the bottle and its artificial contents were offered as the solution for any doubt the mother had, and marketing of these products became more rampant. Members of early mother support groups in a way took the place of the network of family expertise in breastfeeding, and the group became a surrogate grandmother.

The mother and baby get off to a good start when the support from maternity staff and other healthcare professionals complements the support from community breastfeeding support groups and peer counselors. It works best when both are available (Britton et al., 2007). Support to assist the mother to breastfeed her baby needs to start before her baby is born, through breastfeeding-friendly care and education while the mother is pregnant, after she gives birth, and beyond. The very best compliment any of us can give to a health facility is that its care for the breastfeeding mothers who use its services is "seamless."

Instead, all too often the mother experiences conflicting advice, which may leave her confused by the mixed messages. When everyone is working together to support her to breastfeed and everyone around her regards breastfeeding as normal, the mother knows that what she is doing is valued. Provided she has access to information about where she can receive further support, she also knows that she can find someone to listen to her and that she can get *the right advice* at *the right time* from *the right person.*

When I wrote that last sentence, I nearly wrote that it is "ideal" when everyone is working together to support the mother. Then I stopped. "Ideal" implies an aspirational goal. What I want to convey is that this general support for the breastfeeding mother should be normal.

Mother support, however, is not just the mother-to-mother breastfeeding support group. It is not just the health facility and its staff. It is not just the baby's father. The shopkeeper who brings a chair so that the mother can sit and feed her baby at her breast is providing mother support. The passerby who smiles and quietly congratulates her on feeding her baby at the airport or in the shopping mall is also offering mother support, the sort of support that helps her to feel she is doing something normal—which she is. The employer who provides breastfeeding breaks in work time is providing mother support, whether from a commitment to breastfeeding, to retain valued employees, or from the realization that it is an equity issue, especially in a context in which smokers commonly take time out of the workday to go outside, or return late from breaks. The legislators who push through laws to prevent discrimination against a woman on the basis of breastfeeding or who introduce industrial laws that grant longer paid maternity leave and other mother-baby-friendly working conditions—they, also, are providing mother support.

The list is long and space does not allow for a list of every form of mother support possible. New modes of providing support to the breastfeeding mother will surely arise, as has indeed the use of the new technologies. I am not in favor of a long concluding chapter. The chapter authors have provided food for thought with their diverse approaches, which, nevertheless, have some common threads. I urge you, dear reader, to dig into the chapters again and to use this book as a resource, wherever you live and work.

References

AAFP (American Academy of Family Physicians). (2001). *Breastfeeding* (Position Paper). Retrieved April 22, 2006, from http://www.aafp.org/x6633.xml.

AAP (American Academy of Pediatrics Section on Breastfeeding). (2005). Breastfeeding and the use of human milk. *Pediatrics, 115*(2), 496-506.

ABM (Association for Breastfeeding Mothers). (2010). *Welcome to the ABM site.* Retrieved from http://www.abm.me.uk.

Academy for Educational Development (AED) LINKAGES. (2003). *Mother-to-mother support group methodology and breastfeeding and complementary feeding basics.* Curriculum.

Agrasada, G.V. (2005). Postnatal peer counseling for exclusive breastfeeding of low-birthweight infants: A randomized, controlled trial. *Acta Paediatrica, 94,* 1109-15.

Alvarado, R.M., Atalah, E.S., Diaz, S.F., Rivero, S.V., Labbe, M.D., & Escudero, Y.P. (1996). Evaluation of a breastfeeding support programme with health promoter's participation. *Food Nutr Bull, 17,* 49–53.

Amir, L.H., & Donath, S.M. (2008). Socioeconomic status and rates of breastfeeding in Australia: Evidence from three recent national health surveys. *The Medical Journal of Australia, 189*(5), 254-256.

Anderson, A., Damio, G., Young, S., Chapman, D., & Perez-Escamilla, R. (2005). A randomized trial assessing the efficacy of peer counseling on exclusive breastfeeding in a predominantly Latina low-income community. *Archives of Pediatric and Adolescent Medicine, 159*(9), 836-841. doi: 10.1001/archpedi.159.9.836.

Arlotti, J., Cottrell, B., Lee, S., & Curtin, J. (1998). Breastfeeding among low-income women with and without peer support. *Journal of Community Health Nursing, 15*(3), 163-178.

Auer, C. & Gromada, KK. (1998). A case report of breastfeeding quadruplets: Factors perceived as affecting breastfeeding. *Journal of Human Lactation, 14*(2), 135-141.

Australian Breastfeeding Association. (2005). *2005 Annual Report.* Retrieved on 10 July 2010 from http://www.breastfeeding.asn.au/aboutaba/documents/annual.

Australian Bureau of Statistics. (2003). 4810.0.55.001 - Breastfeeding in Australia, 2001. *National Health Survey.* Retrieved 15th August 2006, 2006, from http://www.abs.gov.au/Ausstats/abs@.nsf/525a1b9402141235ca25682 000146abc/8e65d6253e10f802ca256da40003a07c!OpenDocument.

Australian Bureau of Statistics. (2007a). *2006 Census Data - Australia.* Retrieved from http://www.censusdata.abs.gov.au.

Australian Bureau of Statistics. (2007b). *General Social Survey: Summary Results, Australia, 2006* Cat # 4159.0. Retrieved July 23rd 2010, from http://www. abs.gov.au/ausstats/abs@.nsf/mf/4159.0#FINANCIAL%20STRESS%20 AND%20INCOME.

Australian Bureau of Statistics. (2009). *Australian Social Trends, 2008; Education Across Australia.* Cat # 4102.0. Retrieved December 6th 2011, from http:// www.abs.gov.au/AUSSTATS/abs@.nsf/Lookup/4102.0Chapter6002008.

Australian Bureau of Statistics. (2010). *Births, Australia, 2009.* Cat. no. 3301.0. Sydney, NSW: Commonwealth of Australia. Retrieved January 2, 2012 from http://www.ausstats.abs.gov.au/Ausstats/subscriber.nsf/0/10BEDC49AFCA CC1FCA2577CF000DF7AB/$File/33010_2009.pdf.

Australian Health Ministers' Conference. (2009). *The Australian National Breastfeeding Strategy 2010-2015.* Canberra: Australian Government Department of Health and Ageing.

Australian Institute of Family Studies. (2008). *Growing Up In Australia: The Longitudinal Study of Australian Children, Annual Report 2006-07.* Canberra: Department for Families, Housing, Community Services and Indigenous Affairs.

Ball, H.L. (2007). Together or apart? A behavioural and physiological investigation of sleep arrangements for twin babies. *Midwifery, 23*(4), 404-412.

Bandura, A. (1977). Self-efficacy: Toward a unifying theory of behavioral change. *Psychology Reviews, 84*(2), 191-215.

Barona-Vilar, C., Escriba-Aguir, V., & Ferrero-Gandia, R. (2009). A qualitative approach to social support and breast-feeding decisions. *Midwifery, 25*(2), 187-194.

BCCT (Baby Café Charitable Trust). *Annual Reports.* UK: BCCT. Retrieved from http://www.thebabycafe.org/faqs/129-annual-reports.html.

Beck, C.T. (2002a). Releasing the pause button: Mothering twins during the first year of life. *Qualitative Health Research, 12*(5), 593-608.

Beck, C.T. (2002b). Mothering multiples: A meta-synthesis of qualitative research. *MCN: The American Journal of Maternal Child Nursing, 27*(4), 214-221.

Becker, G.E., Cooney, F., & Smith, H.A. (2011). Methods of milk expression for lactating women. *Cochrane Database Sys Rev. Dec 7*; 12, CD006170.

Berlin, C. (2007). "Exclusive" breastfeeding of quadruplets. *Breastfeeding Medicine, 2*(2), 125-126.

Bernaix, L., Schmidt, C., Jamerson, P., Seiter, L., & Smith, J. (2006). The NICU experience of lactation and its relationship to family management style. *Maternal Child Nursing, 31*(2), 95-100. doi: 10.1097/00005721-200603000-00008.

Bhandari, N., Bahi, R., Mazumdar, S., Martines, J., Black, R.E., Bhan, M.K., & Infant Feeding Study Group. (2003). Effect of community based promotion of exclusive breast feeding on diarrheal illness and growth: A cluster randomized controlled trial. *Lancet, 361*, 1418-1423.

Bhutta, Z.A., Ahmed, T., Black R.E, Cousens, S., Dewey, K., Giugliani, E., et al. (2008). What works? Interventions for maternal and child undernutrition and survival. *Lancet, 371*(9610), 417-440.

Black, B.P., Holditch-Davis, D., & Miles, M.S. (2009). Life course theory as a framework to examine becoming a mother of a medically fragile preterm infant. *Research in Nursing & Health, 32*(1), 38-49. doi: 10.1002/nur.20298.

Bland, R.M., Little, K.E., Coovadia, H.M., Coutsoudis, A., Rollins, N.C., & Newell, M.L. (2008). Intervention to promote exclusive breastfeeding for the first 6 months of life in a high HIV prevalence area. *AIDS, 22*, 883-891.

Bland, R., Rollins, N.C., Coovadia, H.M., Coutsoudis, A., & Newell, M.L. (2007). Infant feeding counselling for HIV-infected and uninfected women: Appropriateness of choice and practice. *Bulletin of the World Health Organization, 85*, 289-296.

Blum, L.M., & Vanderwater, E. A. (1993). Mother to mother: A maternalist organization in late capitalist America. *Social Problems, 40*(3), 285-300.

Bolling, K., Grant, C., Hamlyn, B., & Thornton, A. (2007). *Infant feeding 2005.* London: National Health Service.

Bowers, N., & Gromada, K.K. (2006). *Care of the multiple-birth family: Pregnancy and birth* (rev. ed., nursing module). White Plains, NY: March of Dimes.

BPNI/IBFAN. (2009). *The "3 in 1" training program: Capacity building initiative for building health workers' skills in infant and young child feeding counselling training course*. Retrieved from http://www.bpni.org/Training/3-in-1-TP-BPNI.pdf.

Britton, C., McCormick, F.M., Renfrew, M.J., Wade, A., & King, S.E. (2007). Support for breastfeeding mothers. *Cochrane Database of Systematic Reviews, 24*(1): CD001141.

Callen, J., & Pinelli, J. (2005). A review of the literature examining the benefits and challenges, incidence and duration, and barriers to breastfeeding in preterm infants. *Advances in Neonatal Care, 5*(2), 72-88. doi: 10.1016/j.adnc.2004.12.003.

Caplan, G. (1990). Spontaneous and natural support systems. In A.H. Katz, & E.I. Bender (Eds.), *Helping one another: Self-help groups in a changing society*. Oakland, CA: Third Party Publishing.

CDC (Center for Disease Control & Prevention). (2009). Quick stats: Percentage of live births by cesarean delivery, by plurality – United States, 1996, 2000, and 2006. *Morbidity & Mortality Weekly Report, 58*(19), 542. Retrieved January 2, 2012 from http://www.cdc.gov/mmwr/preview/mmwrhtml/mm5819a9.htm.

CDC (Centers for Disease Control and Prevention). 2011. *Breastfeeding report card-United States, 2011*. Retrieved from http://www.cdc.gov/breastfeeding/data/reportcard.htm.

CDC (Centers for Disease Control and Prevention). (2005). *National Immunisation Survey - Table 3: Any and exclusive breastfeeding rates by age, 2005*. Retrieved August 15, 2006, from http://www.cdc.gov/breastfeeding/data/NIS_data/index.htm.

CDC (Centers for Disease Control and Prevention). (2006). *Breastfeeding: Data and statistics: Breastfeeding practices – Results from the 2005 National Immunization Survey*. Retrieved July 28, 2006, from: http://www.cdc.gov/breastfeeding/data/NIS_data/index.htm.

CDC (Centers for Disease Control and Prevention). (2011). *Breastfeeding among U.S. children born 2000-2008, CDC National Immunization Survey*. Retrieved from http://www.cdc.gov/breastfeeding/data/NIS_data/index.htm.

CDC (Centers for Disease Control and Prevention). (2011). *Breastfeeding Report Card - United States 2011*. Atlanta, Georgia. Retrieved December 6th 2011, from http://www.cdc.gov/breastfeeding/data/reportcard.htm.

Chamberlain, L., McMahon, M., Philipp, B., & Merewood, A. (2006). Breast pump access in the inner city: A hospital-based initiative to provide breast pumps for low-income women. *Journal of Human Lactation, 22*(1), 94-98. doi: 10.1177/0890334405284226.

Chapman, D., Damio, G., Young, S., & Perez-Escamilla, R. (2004). Effectiveness of breastfeeding peer counseling in a low-income, predominantly Latina population: A randomized controlled trial. *Archives of Pediatric and Adolescent Medicine, 158*(9), 897-902.

Charchuk, M. & Simpson, C. (2005). Hope, disclosure, and control in the neonatal intensive care unit. *Health Communication, 17*(2), 191-203. doi: 10.1207/s15327027hc1702_5.

Choi, Y., Bishal, D., & Minkovitz, C.S. (2009). Multiple births are a risk factor for postpartum maternal depressive symptoms. *Pediatrics, 123*(4), 1147-1154. Retrieved January 2, 2012 from http://pediatrics.aappublications.org/cgi/content/full/123/4/1147.

Cleveland, L. (2008). Parenting in the neonatal intensive care unit. *Journal of Obstetric, Gynecologic, and Neonatal Nursing, 37*(6), 666-91. doi: 10.1111/j.1552-6909.2008.00288.x.

Coovadia, H.M., Rollins, N.C., Bland, R.M., Little, K., Coutsoudis, A., Bennish, M.L., & Newell, M.L. (2007). Mother-to-child transmission of HIV-1 infection during exclusive breastfeeding: the first six months of life: An intervention cohort study. *Lancet, 369*(9567), 1107-16.

Coutsoudis, A, Coovadia, H.M., & Wilfert, C.M. (2009). Formula-feeding is not a sustainable solution. *Bull World Health Organ, 87*(8), A-B.

Cowan, C. (2011). La Leche League International. In O'Reilly, A., (Ed.) *The 21st Century motherhood movement: Mothers speak out on why we need to change and how to do it* (pp. 207-218). Toronto: Demeter Press.

Cregan M.D., De Mello T.R., Kershaw D., McDougall K., & Hartmann P. E. (2002). Initiation of lactation in women after preterm delivery. Acta Obstetricia Gynecologica Scandinavica, 81(9), 870-877. doi: 10.1034/j.1600-0412.2002.810913.x.

D'Addato, A.V. (2007). Secular trends in twinning rates. Journal of Biosocial *Science, 39*(1), 147-151.

Damato, E.G., Dowling, D.A., Standing, T.S., & Schuster, S.D. (2005a). Explanation for the cessation of breastfeeding in mothers of twins. *Journal of Human Lactation, 21*(3), 296-304.

Damato, E.G., Dowling, D.A., Madigan, E.A., & Thanattherakul, C. (2005b). Duration of breastfeeding for mothers of twins. *Journal of Obstetric, Gynecologic & Neonatal Nursing, 34*(2), 201-209.

Delgadillo, J. L. (2002). Estrategia válida para la lactancia exitosa: IHANM. *Pediatr Py, 29*(1).

Delgadillo, J. L. (2003). Mortalidad Infantil: Propuesta para su reducción. *Pediatria, 30*(2), 35.

Dennis, C.L. (2002). Breastfeeding initiation and duration: A 1990-2000 literature review. *Journal of Obstetric, Gynecologic, and Neonatal Nursing, 31*(1), 12-32. doi:10.1111/j.1552-6909.2002.tb00019.x.

Dennis, C.L., & Faux, S. (1999). Development and psychometric testing of the Breastfeeding Self-Efficacy Scale. *Research in Nursing & Health, 22*(5), 399-409.

Dennis, C.L., Hodnett, E., Gallop, R., & Chalmers, B. (2002). The effect of peer support on breast-feeding duration among primiparous women: A randomized controlled trial. *Canadian Medical Association Journal, 166*(1), 21-28.

Department of Health. (2000). *The NHS plan.* Retrieved from: http://www.dh.gov.uk.

Department of Health (2004). *Good practice and innovation in breastfeeding.* Retrieved from: http://www.dh.gov.uk.

Department of Health. (2010). Infant Mortality National Support Team tackling health inequalities in Infant and Maternal Health Outcomes Report. London: Department of Health.

Department of Health/Department for Children, Schools, and Families. (2009). Commissioning local breastfeeding support services. London: DH/DCSF.

de Verón, L. (Dec. 2003 – Jan. 2004). 20 years of La Liga de la Leche del Paraguay, Lili, Asunción, Paraguay LEAVEN, 39 (6), pp. 137-38.

DGEEC (Dirección General de Estadística, Encuestas y Censos Paraguay (DGEEC) Encuesta Permanente de Hogares). (2010a). *Trípticos EPH 2010, Total País, Asunción y Departamentos.* Retrieved from http://www.dgeec.gov.py/Publicaciones/Biblioteca/EHP2010/Triptico%20EPH%20total%20pais%202010.pdf.

DGEEC. (2010b). Principales Resultados de Pobreza y Distribución del Ingreso, EPH Encuestas Permanente de Hogares, p 5.

Directorate of Town Panchayats. (2010). *Empowerment activities.* Retrieved from http://www.tn.gov.in/dtp/shg.htm.

Division of Child Health and Development. (1998). *Evidence for the ten steps to successful breastfeeding*. World Health Organization, Geneva.

Donath, S.M., & Amir, L.H. (2002). The introduction of breast milk substitutes and solid foods: Evidence from the 1995 National Health Survey. *Australian and New Zealand Journal of Public Health, 26*(5), 481-484.

Donovan, F. (1977). *Voluntary organisations: A case study* (p. 26). Bundoora, Victoria: Preston Institute of Technology Press.

Dykes, F. (2003). Infant feeding initiative: A report evaluating the breastfeeding practice projects 1999-2002. Department of Health.

Dykes, F, (2005). Government funded breastfeeding peer support projects: Implications for practice. *Maternal & Child Nutrition, 1*, 21-31.

Dykes, F., & Griffiths, H. (1998). Societal influences upon initiation and continuation of breastfeeding. *British Journal of Midwifery, 6*(2), 76-80.

Dyson, L., Renfrew, M., McFadden, A., McCormick, F., Herbert, G., & Thomas, J. (2006). *Promotion of breastfeeding initiation and duration: Evidence into practice briefing*. London: National Institute for Health and Clinical Excellence.

Dyson, L., Renfrew, M.J., McFadden, A., McCormick, F., Herbert, G., & Thomas, J. (2010). Policy and public health recommendations to promote the initiation and duration of breast-feeding in developed country settings. *Public Health Nutrition, 13*(1), 137-144.

Ekstrom, A., Widstrom, A.M., & Nissen, E. (2003). Breastfeeding support from partners and grandmothers: Perceptions of Swedish women. *Birth, 30*(4), 261-266.

Emmanuel, E.N., Creedy, D.K., St. John, W., & Brown, C. (2011). Maternal role development: The impact of maternal distress and social support following childbirth. *Midwifery, 27*(2), 265-272. doi: 10.1016/j.j.midw.2009.07.003.

ENDSSR. (2008). Informe Final, (National Survey of Demographic, Sexual and Reproductive Health 2008, Final Report) October 2009, Asuncion, Paraguay, 57-58, 237-239, 278-279. Retrieved from http://pdf.usaid.gov/pdf_docs/PNADR811.pdf.

Ertem, I.O., Votto, N., & Leventhal, J.M. (2001). The timing and predictors of the early termination of breastfeeding *Pediatrics, 1007*, 543 - 548.

EURO-PERISTAT Project. (2008). *European perinatal health report*. Paris, France: Author. Retrieved January 2, 2012 from http://www.europeristat.com/bm.doc/european-perinatal-health-report.pdf.

Fairbank, L., O'Meara, S., Renfrew, M.W., Snowden, A., & Lister-Sharp, D. (2000). A systematic review to evaluate the effectiveness of interventions to promote the initiation of breastfeeding. *Health Technology Assessment, 4*, 1-171.

Fenwick, J., Barclay, L., & Schmied, V. (2001). "Chatting": an important clinical tool in facilitating mothering in neonatal nurseries. *Journal of Advanced Nursing, 33*(5), 583-593. doi: 10.1046/j.1365-2648.2001.01694.x.

Ferguson T., & The e-Patient Scholars Working Group. (2010). *E-Patients: How they can help us heal healthcare.* Retrieved from http://e-patients. net/e-Patients_White_Paper.pdf.

Finn, L.D., Bishop, B.J., & Sparrow, N. (2009). Capturing dynamic processes of change in GROW mutual help groups for mental health. *American Journal of Community Psychology, 44*(3-4), 302.

Fjeldsoe, B.S., Marshall, A.L., & Miller, Y.D. (2009). Behavior change interventions delivered by mobile telephone short message service. *American Journal of Preventative Medicine, 36*(2).

Flacking, R., Ewald, U., Nyqvist, K., & Starrin, B. (2006). Trustful bonds: A key to "becoming a mother" and to reciprocal breastfeeding. Stories of mothers of very preterm infants at a neonatal unit. *Social Science and Medicine, 62*(1), 70-80. doi:10.1016/j.soscimed.2005.05.026.

Fogg, B.J., & Eckles, D. (2007). *Mobile persuasion : 20 perspectives on the future of behavior change.* Standford, CA : Stanford Captology Media.

Foster, K, Lader, D., & Cheesbrough, S. (1995). *Infant feeding 1995.* Great Britain: Office for National Statistics, Social Survey Division.

Fox, N.S., Rebarber, A., Roman, A.S., Klauser, C.K., Peress, D., & Saltzman, D.H. (2010). Weight gain in twin pregnancies and adverse outcomes: Examining the 2009 Institute of Medicine guidelines. *Obstetrics & Gynecology, 116*(1), 100-106. Retrieved January 2, 2012 from http:// journals.lww.com/greenjournal/Fulltext/2010/07000/Weight_Gain_in_ Twin_Pregnancies_and_Adverse.17.aspx#.

Frossell, S. (1998). If 'breast is best' then what is the problem? *British Journal of Midwifery, 6*(5), 316-319.

Furman, L., Wilson-Costello, D., Friedman, H., Taylor H.G., Minich, N., & Hack, M. (2004). The effect of neonatal maternal milk feeding on the neurodevelopmental outcome of very low birth weight infants. *Journal of Developmental and Behavioral Pediatrics, 25*(4), 247–253. doi: 10.1097/00004703-200408000-00004.

Gallegos, D., Russell-Bennett, R., & Previte, J. (2011). An innovative approach to reducing risks associated with infant feeding: The use of technology. *Journal of Nonprofit and Public Sector Marketing*, In press.

Gartner, L.M., Morton J., Lawrence, R.A., Naylor, A.J., O'Hare, D., Schanler, R.J., et al. (2005). Breastfeeding and the use of human milk. *Pediatrics, 155*(2), 496–506. doi: 10.1542/peds.2004-2491.

Geraghty, S.R., Khoury, J.C., & Kalkwarf, H.J. (2005). Human milk pumping rates of mothers of singletons and mothers of multiples. *Journal of Human Lactation, 21*(4), 413-420.

Geraghty, S.R., Pinney, S.M., Sethurman, G., Roy-Chaudbury, A., & Kalkwarf, H.J. (2004). Breast milk feeding rates of mothers of multiples compared to mothers of singletons. *Ambulatory Pediatrics, 4*(3), 226-231.

Glinianaia, S.V., Rankin, J., & Wright, C. (2008). Congenital anomalies in twins: A register-based study. *Human Reproduction, 23*(6), 1306-1311. Retrieved January 2, 2012 from http://humrep.oxfordjournals.org/content/23/6/1306.full.

Goga, A., et al, (2011). Good Start study. Cited by T. Doherty (2011). Breastfeeding in the context of HIV: The South African experience. Retrieved January 1, 2012, from http://www.ruralhealthconference2011.co.za/uploads/6/7/0/8/6708337/hiv_and_infant_feeding_rudasa_plenary._sept_2011.pdf.

Gribble, K.D. (2001). Mother-to-mother support for women breastfeeding in unusual circumstances: A new method for an old model. *Breastfeeding Review, 9*(3), 13-19.

Gribble, K.D. (2008). Long-term breastfeeding: Changing attitudes and overcoming challenges. *Breastfeeding review: professional publication of the Nursing Mothers' Association of Australia, 16*(1), 5.

Gromada, K.K. (2006). Breastfeeding multiples. *New Beginnings, 23*(6), 244-249. Retrieved January 2, 2012 from http://www.llli.org/nb/nbnovdec06p244.html.

Gromada, K.K. (2007). *Mothering multiples: Breastfeeding and caring for twins or more* (rev ed). Schaumburg, IL: La Leche League International.

Gromada, K.K. (2011a). *Mothering multiples: FAQ.* Retrieved January 2, 2012 from http://www.karengromada.com/faq/.

Gromada, K.K. (2011b). *Birth plan for twins.* Retrieved January 2, 2012 from http://www.karengromada.com/for-parents/.

Gromada, K.K., & Bowers, N. (2005). *Care of the multiple-birth family: Birth through early infancy* (rev. ed., nursing module). White Plains, NY: March of Dimes.

Haider, R., Ashworth, A., Kabir, I., & Huttly, S.R.A. (2000). Effect of community-based peer counsellors on exclusive breastfeeding practices in Dhaka, Bangladesh: A randomized controlled trial. *Lancet, 356,* 1643-47.

Haider, R., Islam, A., Hamadani, J., Amin, N.J., Kabir, I., Malek, M.A., et al. (1996). Breastfeeding counselling in a diarrheal disease hospital. *Bull WHO, 74,* 173-179.

Haider, R., Kabir, I., Huttly, S.R., & Ashworth, A, (2002). Training peer counselors to promote and support exclusive breastfeeding in Bangladesh. *Journal of Human Lactation, 18*(1), 7-12.

Haider, R., Rasheed, S., Sanghvi, T.G., Hassan, N., Pachon, H., Islam, S., et al. (2010). Breastfeeding in infancy: Identifying the program-relevant issues in Bangladesh. *International Breastfeeding Journal, 5,* 21.

Hall Moran, V., Edwards, J., Dykes, F., & Downe, S. (2007). A systematic review of the nature of support for breast-feeding adolescent mothers. *Midwifery, 23*(2), 157-171.

Hannula, L., Kaunonen, M., & Tarkka, T.M. (2008). A systematic review of professional support interventions for breastfeeding. *Journal of Clinical Nursing, 17,* 1132-43.

Hanrahan, J. (2000). Breastfeeding after the loss of a multiple. *Leaven, 36*(5), 12. Retrieved January 2, 2012 from http://www.llli.org/llleaderweb/lv/lvoctnov00p102.html.

Healthy People.gov. (2011). *2020 topics & objectives.* Retrieved December 21, 2011, from http://www.healthypeople.gov/2020/topicsobjectives2020/objectiveslist.aspx?topicId=26.

Heermann, J.A., Wilson, M.E., & Wilhelm, P.A. (2005). Mothers in the NICU: Outsider to partner. *Pediatric Nursing, 31*(3), 176-181.

Henderson, L., Kitzinger, J., & Green, J. (2000). Representing infant feeding: Content analysis of British media portrayals of bottle feeding and breast feeding. *British Medical Journal, 321*(7270), 1196-1198.

Hill, P., Aldag, J., & Chatterton, R. (2001). Initiation and frequency of pumping and milk production in mothers of non-nursing preterm infants. *Journal of Human Lactation, 17*(1), 9-13. doi: 10.1177/089033440101700103.

Hill, P.D., Aldag, J.C., Chatterton, R.C., & Zinaman, M. (2005a). Comparison of milk output between mothers of preterm and term infants: The first 6 weeks after birth. *Journal of Human Lactation, 21,* 22-30. doi: 10.1177/0890334404272407.

Hill, P.D., Aldag, J.C., Chatterton, R.C. & Zinaman, M. (2005b). Primary and secondary mediators' influence on milk output in lactating mothers of preterm and term infants. *Journal of Human Lactation, 21,* 138-150. doi: 10.1177/0890334405275403.

Hoddinott, P., & Pill, R. (1999). Qualitative study of decisions about infant feeding among women in east end of London. *BMJ, 318*(7175), 30-34.

Hoddinott, P., & Roisin, P. (1999). Qualitative study of decisions about infant feeding among women in east end of London. *British Medical Journal, 318* (7175), 30-34.

Hoddinott, P., Britten, J., & Pill, R. (2010). Why do interventions work in some places and not others: A breastfeeding support group trial. *Social Science and Medicine, 70,* 769-778.

Hoddinott, P., Kroll, T., Raja, A., & Lee, A.J. (2010). Seeing other women breastfeed: How vicarious experience relates to breastfeeding intention and behavior. *Maternal Health and Nutrition, 6*(2),134-46.

Holditch-Davis, D. & Miles, M.S. (2000). Mothers' stories about their experiences in the neonatal intensive care unit. *Neonatal Network, 19,* 13-21.

Holman, E. (2009). TXTING4HEALTH: The role of the mobile channel in the healthcare industry and in the sphere of public health. *SMq, XV(S1 Supplement),* 30-35.

Hurling, R., Catt, M., DeBoni, M., Fairley, B., Hurst, T., Murray, P., et al. (2007). Using Internet and mobile phone technology to deliver an automated physical activity program: Randomized controlled trial. *Journal of Medical Internet Research, 9,* e7.

Hurst, N., Myatt, A., & Schanler, R. (1998). Growth and development of a hospital-based lactation program and mother's own milk bank. *Journal of Obstetric, Gynecologic, and Neonatal Nursing, 27,* 503-510. doi: 10.1111/j.1552-6909.1998.tb02616.x.

Hurst, N.M., Meier, P.P., Engstrom, J.L., & Myatt, A. (2004). Mothers performing in-home measurement of milk intake during breastfeeding of their preterm infants: Maternal reactions and feeding outcomes. *Journal of Human Lactation, 20,* 178-187. doi: 10.1177/0890334404264168.

Hylander, M., Strobino, D., & Dhanireddy, R. (1998). Human milk feedings and infection among very low birth weight infants. *Pediatrics, 102*, e38. doi: 10.1542/peds.102.3.e38.

Hylander, M., Strobino, D., Pezzullo, J., & Dhanireddy, R. (2001). Association of human milk feedings with a reduction in retinopathy of prematurity among very low birthweight infants. *Journal of Perinatology, 21*, 356-362. doi: 10.1038/sj.jp.7210548.

Ingram, J., Rosser, J., & Jackson, D. (2005). Breastfeeding peer supporters and a community support group: Evaluating their effectiveness. *Maternal & Child Nutrition, 1*(2), 111-118.

Innocenti Declaration on the protection, promotion, and support of breastfeeding. (1990). Retrieved from www.unicef.org/programme/breastfeeding/innocenti. htm.

Innocenti Declaration + 15. (2005). Retrieved from http://innocenti15.net/ declaration.htm.

International Labour Organization (ILO). (1919). *C3 Maternity Protection Convention, 1919.* Retrieved on February 13, 2012, from http://www.ilo. org/ilolex/cgi-lex/convde.pl?C003.

Jelliffe, D.B., & Jelliffe, E.F.P. (1978). *Human milk in the modern world: Psychosocial, nutritional, and economical significance* (pp. 22-23). Oxford: Oxford University Press.

Johnson, A. (2008). Promoting maternal confidence in the NICU. *Journal of Pediatric Health Care, 22*, 254-257. doi: 10.1016/j.pedhc.2007.12.012.

Jones, L., Woodhouse, D., & Rowe, J. (2007). Effective nurse parent communication: A study of parents' perceptions in the NICU environment. *Patient Education and Counseling, 69*, 206-212. doi: 10.1016/j. pec.2007.08.014.

Kashwaha, K.P. (Ed.). (2010). *Reaching the under 2s: Universalising the delivery of nutrition. Intervention in District Lalitpur, Uttar Pradesh.* Gorakhpur, India: Department of Paediatris, BRD Medical College.

Katz, A.H. (2003-2004). Fellowship, helping, and healing: The re-emergence of self-help groups. *International Journal of Self Help & Self Care, 2*(1), 21-33.

Katz, A. H., & Bender, E. I. (1976). *The strength in us: Self-help groups in the modern world* (pp. 9-21, 23-31, 249-258). New York: New Viewpoints.

Katz, A.H., & Bender, E.I. (1990). Self-help and mutual aid in history: Enduring motifs and current trends. In A.H. Katz & E.I. Bender (Eds.), *Helping one another: Self-help groups in a changing world*. Oakland, CA: Third Party Publishing.

Kavanaugh, K., Meier, P., Zimmerman, B., & Mead, L. (1997). The rewards outweigh the effort: Breastfeeding outcomes for mothers of preterm infants. *Journal of Human Lactation, 13*, 15-21. doi: 10.1177/089033449701300111

Kendall-Tackett, K., Cong, Z., & Hale, T.W. (2011). The effect of feeding method on sleep duration, well-being, and postpartum depression. *Clinical Lactation, 2*(2), 22-26. Retrieved January 2, 2012 from http://www.uppitysciencechick.com/kendall-tackett_CL_2-2.pdf.

Khoury, A.J., Moazzem, S.W., Jarjoura, C.M., Carothers, C., & Hinton, A. (2005). Breast-feeding initiation in low-income women: Role of attitudes, support, and perceived control. [Research Support, U.S. Gov't, Non-P.H.S.]. *Womens Health Issues, 15*(2), 64-72.

King, F.S. (1992). *Helping mothers to breastfeed*. Nairobi: African Medical and Research Foundation.

Kistin, N., Abramson, R., & Dublin, P. (1994). Effect of peer counselors on breastfeeding initiation, exclusivity, and duration among low-income urban women. *Journal of Human Lactation, 10*, 11-15. doi: 10.1177/089033449401000121.

Klaus, M., Kennell, J., & Klaus, P. (1993). *Mothering the mother: How a doula can help you have a shorter, easier, and healthier birth*. Reading, MA: Perseus Books.

Kotler, P., & Lee, N.R. (2008). *Social marketing: Influencing behaviors for good* (3rd ed.). Thousand Oaks, California: Sage Publications.

Labbok, M. (2010). Revisiting – Celebrating Innocenti 20 years! *Report of Expanded Global Breastfeeding Partners' Forum*, Penang Malaysia, October.

La Leche League International. (1963). *The womanly art of breastfeeding* (2nd ed). Franklin Park, Illinois: La Leche League International.

La Leche League International (LLLI). (2009). *Tips for breastfeeding twins*. Information sheet no. 10237. Schaumburg, IL: Author.

Langley, C. (1998). Successful breastfeeding: what does it mean? *British Journal of Midwifery, 6*, 5322-5325.

Lawrence, R.A., & Lawrence, R.M. (2011). *Breastfeeding: A guide for the medical profession* (7th ed). Maryland Heights, Missouri: Elsevier/Mosby.

Leite, A.J.M., Puccini, R., Atallah, A., Cunha, A., Machado, M., Capiberibe, A., et al. (1998). Impact on breastfeeding practices promoted by lay counselors: A randomized and controlled clinical trial. *Journal of Clinical Epidemiology, 51*, S10.Leonard, L.G. (2000). Breastfeeding triplets: The at-home experience. *Public Health Nursing, 17*(3), 211-221.

Leonard, L.G. (2003). Breastfeeding rights of multiple birth families and guidelines for health professionals. *Twin Research, 6*(1), 34-45.

Levine, D. (2007). Using technology to promote youth sexual health. In B.J. Fogg & D. Eckles (Eds.), *Mobile persuasion : 20 perspectives on the future of behavior change* (pp. 15-20). Standford, CA: Stanford Captology Media.

Li, R. & Grummer-Stawn, L. (2002). Racial and ethnic disparities in breastfeeding among United States infants: Third national health and nutrition examination survey, 1988-1994. *Birth, 29*, 251-257. doi: 10.1046/j.1523-536X.2002.00199.x.

Lieberman, M.A. (2003-2004). Self-management in online self-help groups for breast cancer patients: Finding the right group, a speculative hypothesis. *International Journal of Self Help & Self Care, 2*(4): 313-328.

Locklin, M. (1995). Telling the world: Low income women and their breastfeeding experiences. *Journal of Human Lactation, 11*, 285-291. doi: 10.1177/089033449501100415.

Lombardo, C., & Skinner, H. (2003-2004). "A virtual hug": Prospects for self-help online. *International Journal of Self-Help & Self Care, 2*(3), 205-218.

Long, D., Funk-Archuleta, M., Geiger, C., Mozar, A., & Heins, J. (1995). Peer counselor program increases breastfeeding rates in Utah Native American WIC population. *Journal of Human Lactation, 11*, 279-284. doi: 10.1177/089033449501100414.

Lupton, D. & Fenwick, J. (2001). "They've forgotten that I'm the mum": Constructing and practicing motherhood in special care nurseries. *Social Science and Medicine, 53*, 1011-1021. doi:10.1016/S0277-9536(00)00396-8.

MacDorman, M., Martin, J., Mathews, T., Hoyert, D., & Ventura, S. (2005). Explaining the 2001-02 infant mortality increase: Data from the linked birth/infant death data set. *International Journal of Health Services, 35*(3), 415-442.

Madara, E.J. (1999-2000). From church basements to world wide web sites: The growth of self-help support groups online. *International Journal of Self Help & Self Care, 1*(1), 37-48.

Maloni, J.A. (2010). Antepartum bed rest for pregnancy complications: Efficacy and safety for preventing preterm birth. *Biological Research for Nursing, 12*(2), 106-124.

Mannan, I., Rahman, S.M., Sania, A., Seraji, H.R., Mahmud, A.B.M., Begum, N., et al. (2008). Can early postpartum home visits by trained community health workers improve breastfeeding of newborns? *Journal of Perinatology, 28,* 632-640.

Marmot, M., Allen, J., Goldblatt, P., Boyce, T., McNeish, D., Grady, M., et al., (2010). Fair society, healthy lives: strategic review of health in England post 2010. UK: The Marmot Review.

Martens, P. (2002). Increasing breastfeeding initiation and duration at a community level: An evaluation of Sagkeeng First Nation's community health nurse and peer counselor programs. *Journal of Human Lactation, 18,* 236-246. doi: 10.1177/089033440201800305.

Martin, J.A., Hamilton, B.E., Sutton, P.D., Ventura, S.J., Matthews, T.J., & Osterman, M.J. (2011). Births: Final data for 2008. *National Vital Statistics Report, 59*(1). Retrieved January 2, 2012 from http://www.cdc.gov/nchs/data/nvsr/nvsr59/nvsr59_01.pdf.

Mathews, T.J., & MacDorman, M.F. (2010). Infant mortality statistics from the 2006 period linked birth/infant death data set. *National Vital Statistics Report, 58*(17). Hyattsville, MD: National Center for Health Statistics. Retrieved March 19, 2012 from http://www.cdc.gov/nchs/data/nvsr/nvsr58/nvsr58_17.pdf.

McInnes, R.J., & Chambers, J.A. (2008). Supporting breastfeeding mothers: Qualitative synthesis. *Journal of Advanced Nursing, 62*(4), 407-427.

McKenna, J.J., & Gettler, L.T. (2007). Mother-infant co-sleeping with breastfeeding in the western industrialized context: A bio-cultural perspective. In TW Hale & PE Hartmann (Eds.), *Textbook of human lactation* (pp. 271-302). Amarillo, Texas: Hale Publishing. Retrieved January 2, 2012 from http://cosleeping.nd.edu/assets/29735/gettler_co_sleep.bio_cultural.pdf.

Mead, L., Chuffo, R., Lawlor-Klean, P., & Meier, P. (1992). Breastfeeding success with preterm quadruplets. *Journal of Obstetric, Gynecologic & Neonatal Nursing, 21*(3), 221-227.

Meier, P., & Engstrom, J. (2007). Evidence-based practices to promote exclusive feeding of human milk in very low-birthweight infants. *NeoReviews, 8,* e467-477. doi:10.1542/neo.8-11-e467.

Meier, P., Engstrom, J., Mangurten, H., Estrada, E., Zimmerman, B., & Kopparthi, R. (1993). Breastfeeding support services in the neonatal intensive care unit. *Journal of Obstetric and Gynecological Nursing, 22,* 338-347. doi: 10.1111/j.1552-6909.1993.tb01814.x.

Meier, P.P., Engstrom, J.L., Mingolelli, S.S., Miracle, D.J. & Kiesling, S. (2004). The Rush Mother's Milk Club: Breastfeeding interventions for mothers with very-low-birth-weight infants. *Journal of Obstetric, Gynecological and Neonatal Nursing, 33,* 164-174. doi: 10.1177/0884217504263280.

Meier, P., Engstrom, J.L., Patel, A.L., Jegier, B.L., & Bruns, N.E. (2010). Improving the use of human milk during and after the NICU stay. *Clinics in Perinatology, 37,* 217–245. doi:10.1016/j.clp.2010.01.013.

Meier, P.P., Engstrom, J.L., Zuleger, J.L., Motykowski, J.E., Vasan, U., Meier, W.A., et al. (2006). Accuracy of a user-friendly centrifuge for measuring creamatocrits in mother's milk in the clinical setting. *Breastfeeding Medicine, 1,* 79-87.doi: 10.1089/bfm.2006.1.79.

Meinzen-Derr, J., Poindexter, B., Wrage, L., Morrow, A.L., Stoll, B., & Donovan, E.F. (2009). Role of human milk in extremely low birth weight infants' risk of necrotizing enterocolitis or death. *Journal of Perinatology, 29,* 57-62. doi: 10.1038/jp.2008.117.

Mercy Corps. (2009). *Mother support group program brief.* Jakarta, April 2009.

Miles, M.S., Burchinal, P., Holditch-Davis, D., Brunssen, S., & Wilson, S.M. (2002). Perceptions of stress, worry, and support in black and white mothers of hospitalized, medically fragile infants. *Journal of Pediatric Nursing, 17,* 82-88. doi: 10.1053/jpdn.2002.124125.

Miracle, D., Meier, P., & Bennett, P. (2004). Mothers' decisions to change from formula to mothers' milk for very-low-birth-weight infants. *Journal of Obstetric, Gynecological and Neonatal Nursing, 33,* 692-703. doi:10.1177/0884217504270665.

Mitra, S.N., Ali, M.N., Islam, S., Cross, A.R., & Saha, T (1994). *Bangladesh Demographic and Health Survey 1993-94.* Dhaka: National Institute of Population Research and Training, Mitra and Associates, and Micro International Inc.

Mitra, S.N., Al-Sabir, A., Cross, A.R., & Jamil, K. (1997) *Bangladesh Demographic and Health Survey, 1996-1997.* Dhaka: National Institute of Population Research and Training (NIPORT), Mitra and Associates, and Macro International Inc.

Mohrbacher, N., & Kendall-Tackett, K.A. (2005). Breastfeeding made simple: Seven natural laws for nursing mothers. Oakland CA: New Harbinger Publications.

Morrow, A., Guerrero, M.L., Shults, J., Calva, J., Lutter, C., Bravo, J., et al. (1999). Efficacy of home-based peer counseling to promote exclusive breastfeeding: A randomized controlled trial. *The Lancet, 353*, 1226-1231. doi:10.1016/S0140-6736(98)08037-4.

Morton, J., Hall, J.Y., Wong, R.J., Thairu, L., Benitz, W.E., & Rhine, W.D. (2009). Combining hand techniques with electric pumping increases milk production in mothers of preterm infants. *Journal of Perinatology 29*(11), 757-764.

Mothers of Supertwins (MOST). (2007). *Supertwin statistics: Breastfeeding.* Retrieved January 2, 2012 from http://www.mostonline.org/facts_breastfeeding.htm.

Motsoaledi, A. (2011, August 23). *Government adopts breastfeeding-only infant feeding policy.* Media statement by the Minister of Health, Dr Aaron Motsoaledi. Retrieved on August 31, 2011, from http://www.doh.gov.za/show.php?id=3045.

Mozingo, J., Davis, M., Droppleman, P., & Merideth, A. (2000). "It wasn't working": Women's experiences with short-term breastfeeding. *The American Journal of Maternal/Child Nursing, 25*, 120-126.

Multiple Births Foundation (MBF) (2011). *Guidance for health professionals on feeding twins, triplets and higher order multiples.* London, England: Author. Retrieved January 2, 2012 from http://www.multiplebirths.org.uk/MBF_Professionals_Final.pdf.

National Breastfeeding Working Group. (1995). Breastfeeding: good practice guidance to the NHS. Department of Health.

National Department of Health, South Africa. (2010). *Clinical Guidelines: PMTCT (Prevention of Mother-to-Child Transmission).* Retrieved on December 31, 2011, from http://www.fidssa.co.za/images/PMTCT_Guidelines.pdf.

National Institute for Health & Clinical Excellence. (2006*). Routine postnatal care of women and their babies.* NICE Clinical Guidance 37. London: NICE.

National Institute of Population Research and Training (NIPORT). (2001). *Bangladesh Demographic and Health Survey 1999-2000.* Dhaka: National Institute of Population Research and Training (NIPORT), Mitra and Associates, and Macro International Inc.

National Institute of Population Research and Training (NIPORT). (2005). *Bangladesh Demographic and Health Survey 2004.* Dhaka: National Institute of Population Research and Training (NIPORT), Mitra and Associates, and Macro International Inc.

National Institute of Population and Training (NIPORT). (2009) *Bangladesh Demographic and Health Survey 2007*. Dhaka: National Institute of Population Research and Training, Mitra and Associates, Macro International.

Nelson, A. (2006). A metasynthesis of qualitative breastfeeding studies. *Journal of Midwifery and Women's Health, 51*(2), e13-e20. doi: 10.1016/j.jmwh.2005.09.011.

NHMRC (National Health and Medical Research Council). (2003). *Dietary guidelines for children and adolescents in Australia*. Canberra: Commonwealth of Australia.

NHS Centre for Reviews and Dissemination (2000). Promoting the initiation of breastfeeding. *Effective Health Care, 6*(2).

Nichols, J., Schutte, N.S., Brown, R.F., Dennis, C.L., & Price, I. (2009). The impact of a self-efficacy intervention on short-term breast-feeding outcomes. *Health Educ Behav, 36*(2), 250-258.

Njå, A. (1965). *Guidance in infant nutrition and infant care*. [Oslo]. [Prepared in 1948 and last revised in 1965 by physician Arne at the request of the Director of Health.]

Nommsen-Rivers, L. A., Chantry, C. J., Cohen, R. J., & Dewey, K. G. (2010). Comfort with the idea of formula feeding helps explain ethnic disparity in breastfeeding intentions among expectant first-time mothers. *Breastfeeding Medicine, 5*(1), 25-33.

Nor, B., Zembi, Y., Daniels, K., Doherty, T., Jackson, D., Ahlberg, B.M., PROMISE-EBF Study Group. (2009). "Peer but not Peer": Considering the context of infant feeding peer counseling in a high HIV prevalence area. *Journal of Human Lactation, 25*, 427-434.

Nyqvist, K., & Engvall, G. (2009). Parents as their infant's primary caregivers in a neonatal intensive care unit. *Journal of Pediatric Nursing, 24*, 153-163. doi:10.1016/j.pedn.2008.07.006.

Obermayer, J.L., Riley, W.T., Asif, O., & Jersino, J.M. (2004). College smoking-cessation using cell phone text messaging. *Journal of American College Health, 53*(2), 71-78.

Ooki, S. (2008). Breast-feeding rates and related maternal and infants' obstetric factors in Japanese twins. *Environmental Health & Preventive Medicine, 13*(4), 187-197.

Organizacion Panamerica de la Salud. (2010). Indicadores Básicos de Salud, Paraguay 2010, Ministerio de Salud Publica y Bienestar Social del Paraguay (Basic Indicators for Health, Ministry of Public Health and Social Wellbeing of Paraguay).

Östlund, A., Nordström, M., Dykes, F., & Flacking, R. (2010). Breastfeeding in preterm and term twins - maternal factors associated with early cessation: A population-based study. *Journal of Human Lactation, 26*(3), 327-329.

Owen, A. (1978). Self-help approaches in healthcare. *Social Alternatives, 1*(2).

Padovani, F.H.P., Linhares, M.B.M., Pinto, I.D., Duarte, G., & Martinez, F.E. (2008). Maternal concepts and expectations regarding a preterm infant. *The Spanish Journal of Psychology, 11*(2), 581-592.

Pardoe, C., & Williams, J. (2000). The Baby Café pilot project evaluation report. Unpublished.

Parker, D., & Williams, N. (2000). Teens and breastfeeding. *Lactation Consultant Series.* La Leche League International.

Parkinson, J., Russell-Bennett, R., & Previte, J. (2010). *The role of mother-centred factors influencing the complex social behaviour of breastfeeding: Social support and self-efficacy.* Paper presented at the Australian and New Zealand Marketing Academy Conference. Retrieved July 15th 2011, from http://anzmac2010.org/proceedings/index.html.

Passyn, K., & Sujan, M. (2006). Self-accountability emotions and fear appeals: Motivating behavior. *The Journal of Consumer Research, 32*(4), 583-589.

Paterson, H. (1986, November). Special appeal closed – affirmation of NMAA. An end to court case and public liability insurance saga. *NMAA Newsletter, 22*, 9, 11.

Pector, E.A. (2004). How bereaved multiple-birth parents cope with hospitalization, homecoming, disposition for deceased, and attachment to survivors. *Journal of Perinatology, 24*(11), 714-722. Retrieved January 2, 2012 from http://www.nature.com/jp/journal/v24/n11/full/7211170a.html.

Pharoah, P.O.D. & Dundar, Y. (2009). Monozygotic twinning, cerebral palsy and congenital anomalies. *Human Reproduction Update, 15*(6), 239-248. Retrieved January 2, 2012 from http://humupd.oxfordjournals.org/content/15/6/639.long.

Preyde, M., & Ardal, F. (2003). Effectiveness of a parent "buddy" program for mothers of very preterm infants in a neonatal intensive care unit. *Journal of the Canadian Medical Association Journal, 168*, 969-973.

Protheroe, L., Dyson, L., Renfrew, M.J., Bull, J., & Mulvihill, C. (2003). *The effectiveness of public health interventions to promote the initiation of breastfeeding.* Leeds: Health Development Agency.

Pryor, K. (1963). *Nursing your baby.* New York: Harper & Row.

Punthmatharith, B., Buddharat, U. & Kamlangdee, T. (2007). Comparison of needs, need responses, and need response satisfaction of mothers of infants in neonatal intensive care units. *Journal of Pediatric Nursing, 22*(6), 498-506. doi: 10.1016/j.pedn.2006.05.015.

Quinn, V.J. (2005). Improving breastfeeding practices on a broad scale at the community level: Success stories from Africa and Latin America. *Journal of Human Lactation, 21*(3), 345-354.

Raine, P. (2003). Promoting breastfeeding in a deprived area: The influence of a peer support initiative. *Health and Social Care in the Community, 11,* 463-469. doi: 10.1046/j.1365-2524.2003.00449.x.

Raphael, D. (1981). The midwife as doula: A guide to mothering the mother. *Journal of Nurse-Midwifery, 26*(6), 13-15.

Reid, T. (2000). Maternal identity in preterm birth. *Journal of Child Health Care, 4,* 23-29. doi: 10.1177/136749350000400104.

Reiger, K. M. (2001). *Our bodies, our babies: The forgotten women's movement.* Melbourne: Melbourne University Press.

Renfrew, M.J., Dyson, L., Wallace, L., D'Souza, L., McCormick, F., & Spiby, H. (2005*).* The effectiveness of public health interventions to promote the duration of breastfeeding: systematic reviews of the evidence. London: NICE.

Rossman, B., Engstrom, J.L., Meier, P.P., Vonderheid, S.C., Norr, K.F., & Hill, P.D. (2011). "They've walked in my shoes": Mothers of very low birth weight infants and their experiences with breastfeeding peer counselors in the neonatal intensive care unit. *Journal of Human Lactation, 27,* 14-24. doi: 10.1177/0890334410390046.

Rothschild, M.L. (1999). Carrots, sticks and promises: A conceptual framework for the management of public health and social issue behaviors. *Journal of Marketing, 63,* 24-37.

Royal Australian College of Physicians (2006). *Paediatric policy - Breastfeeding.* Retrieved from http://www.racp.edu.au/page/policy-and-advocacy/paediatrics-and-child-health.

Rush Mothers' Milk Club. (n.d.) *In Your Hands* (video). Retrieved October 9, 2011 from http://www.rushmothersmilkclub.com.

Rush Mothers' Milk Club. (2008). *Welcome to the Rush Mothers' Milk Club* [Brochure]. Chicago, IL: Rush University Medical Center.

Saint, L., Maggiore, P., & Hartmann, P. (1986). Yield and nutrient content of milk in eight women breast-feeding twins and one woman breast-feeding triplets. *British Journal of Nutrition, 56*(1), 49-58. Retrieved January 2, 2012 from http://journals.cambridge.org/action/displayAbstract?fromPage=online &aid=874236.

Schafer, E., Vogel, M., Viegas, S., & Hausafus, C. (1998). Volunteer peer counselors increase breastfeeding duration among low-income women. *Birth, 25*, 101-106. doi: 10.1046/j.1523-536x.1998.00101.x.

Schanler, R., Lau, C., Hurst, N., & Smith, E. (2005). Randomized trial of donor human milk versus preterm formula as substitutes for mothers' own milk in the feeding of extremely premature infants. *Pediatrics, 116*, 400-406. doi: 10.1542/peds.2004-1974.

Schanler, R., Shulman, R., & Lau, C. (1999). Feeding strategies for premature infants: Beneficial outcomes of feeding fortified human milk versus preterm formula. *Pediatrics, 103*, 1150-1157. doi: 10.1542/peds.103.6.1150.

Scott, J. A., & Mostyn, T. (2003). Women's experiences of breastfeeding in a bottle-feeding culture. *Journal Human Lactation, 19*(3), 270-277.

Semega-Janneh, I.J. (2005). The Abraham Horwitz Lecture. Breastfeeding: From biology to policy. United Nations Standing Committee on Nutrition (UNSCN). Retrieved from http://www.unscn.org/files/Awards/Horwitz_ Lectures/2nd_lecture_Breastfeeding_from_biology_to_policy.pdf

Shapiro, J.R., Bauer, S., Hamer, R.M., Kordy, H., Ward, D., & Bulik, C.M. (2008). Use of text messaging for monitoring sugar-sweetened beverages, physical activity, and screen time in children: A pilot study. *Journal of Nutrition Education and Behavior, 40*(6), 385-391.

Shaw, E., & Kaczorowski, J. (1999). The effect of a peer counseling program on breastfeeding initiation and longevity in a low-income rural population. *Journal of Human Lactation, 15*, 19-23. doi: 10.1177/089033449901500108.

Shin, H., & White-Traut, R. (2007). The conceptual structure of transition to motherhood in the neonatal intensive care unit. *Journal of Advanced Nursing, 58*, 90-98. doi: 10.1111/j.1365-2648.2006.04194.x.

Sikorski, J., Renfrew, M. J., Pindoria, S., & Wade, A. (2003). Support for breastfeeding mothers: A systematic review. *Paediatric and Perinatal Epidemiology, 17*(4), 407-417.

Sisk, P.M., Lovelady, C.A., Dillard, R.G., Gruber, K. J., & O'Shea, T.M. (2009). Maternal and infant characteristics associated with human milk feeding in very low birth weight infants. *Journal of Human Lactation, 25*, 412-419. doi: 10.1177/0890334409340776.

Smibert, J. (1989). Postnatal care in the 20th century. *Australian Family Physician, 18*(5), 499-503.

Spatz, D. (2004). Ten steps for promoting and protecting breastfeeding for vulnerable infants. *Journal of Perinatal and Neonatal Nursing, 18*, 385-396.

Statistics Canada (2005). Breastfeeding Practices. *Health Reports, 16*(2), 23-31.

Statistics Canada (2008). *Canadian Community Health Survey.* Retrieved August 23, 2009, from http://www.statcan.gc.ca/cgi-bin/imdb/p2SV.pl?Function=ge tSurvey&SurvId=3226&SurvVer=0&InstaId=15282&InstaVer=4&SDDS=3 226&lang=en&db=IMDB&dbg=f&adm=8&dis=2#b3.

Statistics Canada, Minister of Industry. (2009). *Births 2007* (Catalogue no. 84F0210X). Ottawa, Ontario: Author. Retrieved March 19, 2012 from http://dsp-psd.pwgsc.gc.ca/collection_2009/ statcan/84F0210X/84f0210x2007000-eng.pdf.

Statistics South Africa. (2010). *Mortality and causes of death in South Africa, 2008: Findings from death notification.* Statistical release P0309.3 Pretoria: StatsSA. Retrieved August 2011, from http://www.statssa.gov.za/ publications/P03093/P030932008.pdf.

Szucs, K.A., Axline, S.E., & Rosenman, M.B. (2009). Quintuplets and a mother's determination to provide human milk: It takes a village to raise a baby—how about five? *Journal of Human Lactation, 25*(1), 79-84.

Szucs, K.A., Axline, S.E., & Rosenman, M.B. (2010). Induced lactation and exclusive breast milk feeding of adopted premature twins. *Journal of Human Lactation, 26*(3), 309-313.

Tang, Y., Ma, C.X., Cui, W., Chang, V., Ariet, M., Morse, S.B., Resnick, M.B., & Roth, J. (2006). The risk of birth defects in multiple births: A population-based study. *Maternal & Child Health Journal, 10*(1), 75-81. Retrieved September 16, 2011, from http://mch.peds.ufl.edu/recent_pubs/tang_risk_ of_birth_defects_in_multiple_births.pdf.

Tanguay, S., & Heywood, P. (2007). MyFoodPhone: The start of a mobile health revolution. In B.J. Fogg & D. Eckles (Eds.), *Mobile persuasion: 20 perspectives on the future of behavior change* (pp. 21-27). Standford, CA: Stanford Captology Media.

Thorley, V. (1983). NMAA as a self-help organisation. *Breastfeeding Review, 1*(2): 37-39.

Thorley, V. (1990). The Nursing Mothers' Association of Australia as a self-help organization. In A.H. Katz & E.I. Bender (Eds.), *Helping one another: Self-Help groups in a changing world* (pp. 225-233). Oakland, California: Third Party Publishing.

Thorley, V. (2006). Online materials provided to public by mother-support groups in breastfeeding: Observations on readability and access. *International Journal of Self Help & Self Care, 4*(1): 69-77.

Thorley, V. (2009). *Mother to Mother: The History of the Queensland Branch of the Australian Breastfeeding Association.* Coorparoo, Queensland: Queensland Branch of ABA.

Thorley, V. (2011a). The dilemma of breastmilk feeding. *Breastfeeding Review, 19*(1), 5-7.

Thorley, V. (2011b). Middle-class mothers as activists for change: The Australian Breastfeeding Association. In A. O'Reilly (Ed.), *The 21st century motherhood movement: Mothers speak out on why we need to change and how to do it.* Toronto: Demeter Press, (pp. 219-232).

UK Department of Health. (2003). *Infant feeding recommendation.* Retrieved from http://www.dh.gov.uk/en/Publicationsandstatistics/Publications/PublicationsPolicyAndGuidance/DH_4097197.

UNICEF. (1991). *Take the baby-friendly initiative.* New York: UNICEF.

UNICEF. (2011). UNICEF 2010 Annual Reports – Paraguay. Retrieved from http://www.unicef.org/about/annualreport/index_index.html.

UNICEF UK Baby Friendly Initiative. (2009). *Developing a breastfeeding strategy.* UK: UNICEF.

Uraizee, F., & Gross, S. (1989). Improved feeding tolerance and reduced incidence of sepsis in sick very low birthweight (VLBW) infants fed maternal milk [abstract]. *Pediatric Research, 25*, 298A.

USDHHS (United States Dept of Health and Human Services). (2000). *HHS Blueprint for action on breastfeeding:* U.S. Dept of Health and Human Services: Office on Women's Health.

USDHHS (U.S. Department of Health and Human Services) (2011). *The Surgeon General's call for action to support breastfeeding.* Washington, DC: U.S. Department of Health and Human Services. Office of the Surgeon General. Available from http://www.surgeongeneral.gov/topics/breastfeeding/calltoactiontosupportbreastfeeding.pdf.

U.S. Department of Labor. (2010). Break Time for Nursing Mothers provision. *Patient Protection and Affordable Care Act (PPACA)*. Retrieved on November 27, 2011, from http://www.dol.gov/whd/nursingmothers/Sec7rFLSA_btnm. htm.

Vickers, M.C. (2009). *Mother support for breastfeeding: Selected statements and excerpts about mother support in key international documents.* Penang: World Alliance for Breastfeeding Action. Retrieved from http://www.waba.org.my/ pdf/Catalogue.pdf.

Vitaliano, P.P., Russo, J., Carr, J.E., Maiuro, R.D., & Becker, J. (1985). The ways of coping checklist: Revision and psychometric properties. *Multivariate Behavioral Research, 20,* 3-26.

Vohr, B., Poindexter, B., Dusick, A., McKinley, L., Wright, L., Langer, J., et al. (2006). Beneficial effects of breast milk in the neonatal intensive care unit on the developmental outcome of extremely low birth weight infants at 18 months of age. *Pediatrics, 118,* e115-e123. doi: 10.1542/peds.2005-2382.

WABA. (2001). Internal e-dialogue on the Global Initiative for Mother Support (GIMS), 2001. Retrieved from http://www.waba.org.my/whatwedo/gims/ gimsstatement.htm.

WABA. (2002a). GIMS Statement (2002). Retrieved from http://www.waba.org. my/whatwedo/gims/gims+5.htm.

WABA. (2002b). Nurturing the future. Challenges to breastfeeding in the 21st century—WABA Global Forum II Report. Penang: WABA, p. 3.

WABA. (2006). Internal Reports on The Community Seed grants project. Unpublished.

WABA. (2007a). E-dialogue [online summary.] Retrieved from http://www.waba. org.my/whatwedo/gims/gimsstatement.htm.

WABA (2007b). Global Initiative for Mother Support (GIMS), 2007. Retrieved from http://www.waba.org.my/whatwedo/gims/gims+5.html.

WABA. (2007c). GIMS+5 brochure. Retrieved from http://www.waba.org.my/ whatwedo/gims/gimsstatement.htm.

WABA. (2008). WBW 2008 Action Folder. Retrieved on February 13, 2012, from http://www.worldbreastfeedingweek.net/wbw2008/index.htm.

WABA-LLLI. (2007). The state of the art of mother support summit— Breastfeeding mother—Yesterday, today, tomorrow. Retrieved from http:// www.waba.org.my/whatwedo/gims/mssummit2007.htm.

Welsh, S.R. (2011). Breastfeeding twins with confidence. *New Beginnings, 36*(3), 7. Retrieved January 2, 2012 from http://viewer.zmags.com/publication/946 b8eeb#/946b8eeb/8.

West, D. & Marasco, L. (2008). *The breastfeeding mother's guide to making more milk*. NYC: McGraw-Hill.

WHO. (1981). *International code of marketing of breastmilk substitutes* and all subsequent WHA resolutions. Geneva: World Health Organization. Retrieved from http://www.who.int/nutrition/publications/code_english.pdf.

WHO. (1993). *Breastfeeding counselling: a training course*. Geneva: WHO. Retrieved from http://www.who.int/maternal_child_adolescent/documents/who_cdr_93_3/en/index.html.

WHO/UNICEF (1989). *Protecting, promoting, and supporting breastfeeding: The special role of maternity services: A Joint WHO/UNICEF Statement*. Geneva: WHO.

WHO/UNICEF. (1991). *Baby-Friendly Hospital Initiative*. Retrieved from http://www.who.int/nutrition/topics/bfhi/en/index.html.

WHO/ UNICEF (2003). *Global strategy for infant and young child feeding*. Geneva: World Heath Organization / UNICEF. Retrieved from http://www.who.int/nutrition/publications/infantfeeding/9241562218/en/index.html.

WHO/UNICEF. (2009). *Baby-Friendly Hospital Initiative—revised, updated, and expanded for integral care*. Retrieved from http://www.who.int/nutrition/publications/infantfeeding/9789241594950/en/index.html.

WHO/UNICEF (2010). *Countdown to 2015: Decade report (2000-2010): Taking stock of maternal, newborn and child survival*. Annex A. Geneva: WHO. Retrieved December 31, 2011, from http://www.countdown2015mnch.org/documents/2010report/Profile SouthAfrica.pdf.

Wikipedia. (2011). *Cape Town*. Retrieved from http://en.wikipedia.org/wiki/Cape_Town.

Wituk, S., Ealey, S., Brown, L., Shepherd, M., & Meissen, G. (2005). Assessing the needs and strengths of self-help groups: Opportunities to meet healthcare needs. *International Journal of Self Help & Self Care, 3*(1-2): 103-116.

World Bank. (2009). *World Development Indicators 2009*. Retrieved from http://data.worldbank.org/indicator/IT.CEL.SETS.P2.

Yezingane Network & UNICEF (2011). Infant feeding in the context of HIV in South Africa. Revised July 2011. South Africa: Yesingane Network.

Yokoyama, Y., Wada, S., Sugimoto, M., Katayama, M., Saito, M., & Sono, J. (2006). Breastfeeding rates among singletons, twins and triplets in Japan: A population-based study. *Twin Research & Human Genetics. 9*(2), 298-302.

Index

A

Accessibility 212
Advertising Meetings 85
Advocacy 147
Aggressive Marketing Strategies 147
Alive & Thrive project 109
American Academy of Pediatrics 51
Ammehjælpen 65
Ammehjelpen 19, 38, 64, 136
Ammehjelpers 68
Amningshjälpen 64, 136
Annelies Allain 73
Ante-Natal Education 60
Anwar Fazal 73
Anxiety-Nursing-Failure Cycle 24
Association of Breastfeeding Mothers
    57, 117
Australia 21, 183
Australian Breastfeeding Association
    (ABA) 19, 38, 57, 59, 136,
    183, 189, 214
Australian National Health and
    Medical Research Council 55

B

Baby Café 20, 111, 115, 212, 213
Baby Café Local 41, 117
Baby Care Rooms 60
Baby Food Industry 147
Baby-Friendly Health Initiative
    (BFHI) 13
Baby-Friendly Hospital Initiative
    (BFHI) 13, 28, 101, 122, 133,
    195
Baby-Friendly Hospitals 66, 75, 80,
    89
Baby-Friendly Initiative (BFI) 13
Bangladesh 20, 101
Bangladesh Demographic Health
    Surveys (BDHS) 101
Bangladesh Rural Advancement
    Committee 109
Barriers 73, 90, 118, 140, 159, 163,
    216

Barriers to Mother Support 20
Becoming Known 211
Betty Wagner 45
Brand 20, 188, 214
Breastfeeding Advocates 218
Breastfeeding Advocates Network 75
Breastfeeding and Reproductive Issues
    141
Breastfeeding Breaks 31, 139, 221
Breastfeeding Counseling Course, 40
    Hour 103
Breastfeeding Counselors 24, 72
Breastfeeding Fair 97
Breastfeeding-Friendly Care 220
Breastfeeding Information Bureau 75
Breastfeeding in Public 25, 138
Breastfeeding Network 117
Breastfeeding Pamphlets 81
Breastfeeding Peer Counselor-New
    Mother Relationship 160
Breastfeeding Peer Counselors 159
Breastfeeding Promotion Network of
    India (BPNI) 200
Breastfeeding Support Groups for
    Multiples 178
Breastmilk Donors 97
Breast Pumps 159, 163
Business Community 145

C

Campaign for the Protection,
    Promotion, and Support for
    Breastfeeding (CPPBF) 101
Capacity-Building Activities 124
Cesarean Birth Rate 87
Challenges 84, 108
Cincinnati LLL Multiples 182
Circles of Support 26, 153
Clinical Guidelines\
    Prevention of Mother-to-Child
        Transmission 209
Club de Lactante (breastfeeding club)
    96
Code of Ethics 60

Code of Ethics on Infant Formula
    Products 75
Codex Alimentarius Committee 75
Collecting and Storing Milk 159
Comisión Nacional de Fomento de la
    Lactancia Materna
    (COFOLAM) 89
Commercial Influences 29
Communication and Education 161
Community-Based Support 117
Community-Level Mother Support
    197
Community Outreach 86
Compensation 75
Complementary Feeding 97
Conflicting Advice 159, 220
Consistent Message 162
Cost Cutting 215
Counseling\
    A Training Course 74
Cultural Context 58
Cultural Norm 32
Custody/Visitation 29

D

Denmark 65
Derrick and Patrice Jelliffe 38
Developing a Brand 188
Diploma 82
Disciplinary Committee on the Code
    of Ethics 75
Divorce 29
Donated Breastmilk 82
Drop-In Centers 20, 213
Drop-In Support Group 113

E

e-Dialogue 146
Edwina Froehlich 45
Elisabet Helsing 38
Email Counseling 40, 60, 216
Emergencies 32, 125, 153
Emergency Nutrition Network 32
Evaluating Community Support 197
Evidence-Based Material 67
Evidence-Based Technology and
    Resources 161

Exclusive Breastfeeding 55, 97, 102,
    104, 105, 107, 134, 196, 197,
    206
Expatriate 81, 216
Expatriate Members 73
Extended Families 35

F

Facebook 40, 58, 75, 85
Face-to-Face Counseling 60, 84
Face-to-Face Group 38
Face-to-Face Support 185
Family 71
Fathers 17, 30, 84, 107, 125, 143,
    144, 145, 152, 220
Father Support Groups 144
Feminist Movement 68
Financial Sustainability 211, 213
Five Circles of Support 153
Focus Group Discussions 105
Food Security and Labeling
    Committee 75
Free Community Announcements
    212
Funding 89, 94, 104, 108, 115, 147,
    206
Fundraising 71, 213

G

Generating Income 214
Ghana 121
GIMS 137, 145
GIMS+5 Statement 149
Global Initiative for Father Support
    (GIFS) 142
Global Network 137
Global Strategy for Infant and Young
    Child Feeding 55, 134
Goals of the GIMS+5 149
Government Policies 19
Government Support 139
Grandmothers 26, 30, 37, 91, 122,
    125, 143
Grants 215
Groote Schuur Hospital 204
Guarani 82

H

Hand Express 94, 97

Hand Expression 18
Healthcare Provider 28
Health Professional Education 60
Health Professional-Led Model 115
Health Professionals 16, 30, 69, 73,
        81, 98, 115, 147, 176, 184,
        208, 218, 220
Health Services 139
Healthy People 2020 Goals 31
HIV/AIDS 207, 209
HIV and AIDS Support Groups 149
HIV and Infant Feeding Policies 150
Home Visits 72, 84
Hospital Cruz Roja Paraguaya (Red
        Cross Paraguay) 82, 90
Hospital-Grade Pumps 18
Hospital Practices 147
Hospital Visits 72
Human Milk Bank 95
Human Milk Feedings 157
Human Rights 142

I

IBCLC Support 66
Improve Hospital Practices 93
Inclusiveness 211, 213
In-Depth Interviews 105
India 199
Indigenous Population 88
Infant and Young Child Feeding
        (IYCF) 196
Infant and Young Child Feeding
        Promoters 109
Information Dissemination 148
Innocenti Declaration 13, 134, 196
International Baby Food Action
        Network (IBFAN) 73, 200
International Board Certified Lactation
        Consultants 30
International Childrens' Day
        Celebration 73
International Code of Marketing of
        Breastmilk Substitutes 102
International Code of Marketing of
        Breast-Milk Substitutes 13, 29
International Labor Organization
        (ILO) 31
International Organisation for
        Consumer Union (IOCU) 73
International Organizations 121, 122

International Policies 134
International Stakeholders 147
Internet 85
Internet Forum 60

J

Jakarta, Indonesia 122

K

Kangaroo Mother Care 178

L

Lack of Accurate Information 147
Lactancia Materna (Breastfeeding Fair)
        95
La Leche League 19, 45, 81, 117,
        172, 218
La Leche League International 59,
        135
La Leche League International Child
        Survival Project in Honduras
        123
La Leche League International Peer
        Counselor Program 206
La Leche League of Paraguay (LLLPy)
        19
La Liga de Leche Materna del Paraguay
        (LLLPy) 81
Lalitpur Project 16, 199
Language Differences 82, 216
Language, Guarani 87
Language, Jopará 87
Legislation 28, 138, 139
Legislators 221
Libraries 72
Listening-Dialoguing-Acting Skills
        129
LLL Leaders 81, 84, 87, 91, 93
Local Group Meetings 60
Longitudinal Survey of Australian
        Children 183
Low-Income and African-American
        Mothers 163

M

Malaysia 71, 216
Malaysian Breastfeeding Association
        71

Malaysian Council for Child Welfare (MCCW) 73, 74
Malaysian Trade Union Congress 74
Male Peer Counselors 16, 21, 87, 205, 208
Maori and Pacific Islander mothers 218
Marian Tompson 45, 50
Mary Ann Cahill 45
Mary Ann Kerwin 45
Mary Paton 38
Mary White 45
Maternity Care Practices 30
Maternity Leave 32, 59, 72, 221
Maternity Protection Campaign 74
Maternity Protection Legislation 66
Maternity Ward Visits 82
Medical Establishment 49
Membership Subscriptions 214
Mentors 67, 73, 200
Mercy Corps 122, 124
Midwife Obstetric Units 204
Milk Club Taxi 164
Mobile Devices 21, 193
Mobile Phone Networks 183
Mobile Phones 99, 186, 193
Monitoring 31, 80, 89, 104, 107, 118, 124, 145, 169, 193, 200
Moral Support 139
Mother Baby-Friendly Hospital Initiative (MBFHI) 13
Mothering the Mother 169
Mother of Twins (MOT) 172
Mother's Club 93
Mother's Confidence 24, 46
Mother's Milk Club 17
Mothers of Twins/Mothers of Multiples (MOT/MOM) 173
Mother Support 15, 23, 66, 142, 219, 220
Mother Support Groups 43, 56, 80, 89, 90, 123, 133, 148, 197, 211
Mother Support Map 152
Mother Support Summit 145, 152
Mother-to-Mother Support 18
Mother-to-Mother Support Groups 16, 65, 121, 140, 146, 182, 197
Mother-to-Mother Support Group Training 124

Mother-to-Mother Support (MtMS) Groups 66
Mother-to-Mother Support (MTMS) Task Force 134
Motivators 123
Movement 65, 66
MSTF e-Newsletter 143, 154
m-Technologies 186
Multiples, Birth Support 177
Multiples, Breastfeeding Support Group Meetings 180
Multiples, Do's and Don'ts 181
Multiples, Internet Support Groups 182
Multiples, Maternal Complications 175
Multiples, Mothers of 21, 39
Multiples, Postnatal Support 178
Multiples, Sleep Deprivation 179
Multiples-Specific Resources 176
Multiples, Support During Pregnancy 176
MumBubConnect 188
MumBubConnect, Lessons Learned 192
MumBubConnect (MBC) Program 183
MumBubConnect, Process Evaluation 192

N

National Breastfeeding Consultative Meeting 208
National Breastfeeding Helpline 60
National Breastfeeding Strategies 61
National Campaign 30
National Congress Women's Organisation 74
Nationally Recognized Qualifications in Breastfeeding Education 60
Natural Childbirth and Parenting Groups 141
Natural Disasters 25, 32
Natural Parenting\ Father Support Group 75
NCT Group 116
neonatal intensive care unit 157
newsletter 40, 143
New Zealand 20, 217
NGOs 121, 122

Norway 64
Nursing Mothers' Association of
      Australia 19
Nursing Mothers' Council 38
Nutritional Support 139

O

Online Breastfeeding Mothers of
      Multiples Support Group 182
On-Line Breastfeeding Support
      Groups 75
Online Consultative Dialogue 152
On-Line Discussion 137
Online Discussion Forums 186
Online Groups 39
Online Resources 135
Optimize Milk Output 162

P

Pakistan 145
Paraguay 79, 216
Parent-Focused Information Packets
      and Handouts 168
Parhupar (Parto Humanizado
      Paraguay) 87
Pediatricians 81, 90, 93
Peer Counseling 20, 30, 56, 88, 102,
      124, 154, 185, 198
Peer Counseling Program 102
Peer Counseling Program 205
Peer Counselor Program 20
Peer Counselor Responsibilities 165
Peer Counselors 16, 89, 94, 103, 107,
      146, 198, 204
Peer Support Groups 197
Persatuan Penasihat Penyusuan Ibu
      Malaysia (PPPIM) 19, 71
Physical Challenges, Babies 217
Policy 28, 146, 184, 209
Pregnant Adolescents 86
Pregnant Teens 92
Prevention of Mother to Child
      Transmission (PMtCT) 207
Printed Information 40
Problem-Owners 66
Projects vs Movements 65
Publications 47, 60, 67
Public Policy 28

R

Recruiting Women 189
Red Amamanta Paraguay 98
Referral to Mother Support 17
Reproductive Cycle 141, 142
Reproductive Rights 142
Role Models 164
Room-in 72
Rush Mother's Club Luncheons 162
Rush Mothers' Milk Club (RMMC)
      16, 20, 157, 212

S

Scandinavia 63
School for Mothers and Future
      Mothers 87
Self-Confidence 124
Self-Help Group 19, 37
Self-Help Movement 35
Self-Sustainability 37, 218
Share Experiences 42, 91
Short-Message-Service (SMS) Program
      183
Social Change 66
Social Marketing Program 183, 187
Social Media 21, 186
Social Network 28, 57
South Africa 21, 203
Staff Availability and Turnover 108
Stay-at-Home Mothers 84
Sticker, Breaastfeeding Welcome Here
      60
Stories 122, 167
Storytelling 20, 122, 206, 219
Sudanese Breastfeeding Association
      (SABA) 145
Supervision 104, 107, 115, 125, 199
Support, Family 27, 117, 149
Support Networks 103, 139
Surgeon General's Call to Action to
      Support Breastfeeding 29
Sweden 64

T

Technological Innovations 27
Technology 35, 89, 162, 173, 183,
      215
Telephone Counseling 40
Telephone Help 84

Ten Steps to Successful Breastfeeding 13
Text Messaging 183
The Global Initiative for Mother Support (GIMS) for Breastfeeding 137
The Ministry of Public Health and Social Welfare MSPBS 88
The Womanly Art of Breastfeeding 48
Trained Volunteer Breastfeeding Counselor 60
Training 16, 28, 30, 41, 56, 60, 72, 90, 98, 101, 107, 121, 144, 164, 184, 205, 215
Training and Assistance for Health & Nutrition (TAHN) Trust 104
Training Modules 72
Training Program 200
Training Workshops 91
Twins 16, 171
Two-Way SMS Text Messaging Service 187
Types of Support 26

U

UNICEF 73, 89, 90, 98, 126, 147, 198, 205
UNICEF Community IYCF Counselling Package 126
Unidads de Salud de la Familia (USF) 97
United Kingdom 111
United States 20, 157, 173

V

Village Level Counselors 200
Viola Lennon 45
Volunteers 15, 116, 211, 216
Volunteer Service 75
Volunteer Workforce 61

W

WABA Mother Support Task Force (MSTF) 143, 154
War 32
Website 40, 60, 85, 115, 144, 154, 185, 217
Weekly Text Messages 190
Wellstart 73
Wellstart Training Curriculum 206
Western Cape Department of Health 203
WHO 73
WHO Counseling Course 103
Woman's Right to Breastfeed 29
Word of Mouth 47, 71
Working Mothers 72, 91, 138, 147
Workplace Policies 31
World Alliance for Breastfeeding Action (WABA) 16, 25, 74, 104, 134
World Bank 104, 147
World Breastfeeding Week 26, 74, 90, 97, 136, 148, 152
World Health Assembly Resolutions 29
World Health Organization 81, 101, 209

About the Editors

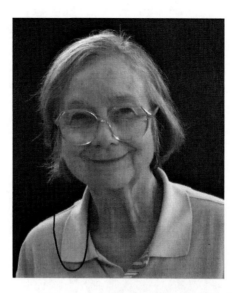

Virginia Thorley. Photo by Lesley McBurney.

Virginia became interested in mother support when she was the recipient of the *right advice* from the *right person* at the *right time* as a new mother in 1965. She was living in a remote area of Queensland, Australia, and had given birth in a provincial city where consistently deleterious advice on breastfeeding had resulted in iatrogenic lactation failure. Before the birth, La Leche League's Marian Tompson had provided her with advice by letter and an article about relactation (resuming breastfeeding) in case of a bad start. When Virginia returned home with a baby who was receiving her total calculated intake in the form of artificial baby milk by bottle, La Leche League (LLL's) manual, *The Womanly Art of Breastfeeding*, had arrived and she immediately applied the two pages on relactation. Four and a half days later, her baby's intake was entirely breastmilk. Believing that other mothers needed accurate advice and support, in 1966 Virginia qualified as a Leader with LLL and then with the Australian Breastfeeding Association (then the Nursing Mothers' Association).

Virginia was in the initial cohort to certify IBCLC in 1985 and is certified to 2016. She is the author of *Successful Breastfeeding* (several editions, Australia, 1974-1991), *Feeding Your Baby and Young Child in Australia* (1984, 2nd edition issued as *Feeding Baby and Child*, 1992), *Establishing Breastfeeding* (1989), and *Mother to Mother: The History of the Queensland Branch of the Australian Breastfeeding Association* (2009). Her chapter on the Australian Breastfeeding Association appeared in the Demeter Press book on the 21st century motherhood movement (2011). A hospital assessor and educator for the Baby-Friendly Health Initiative (BFHI), Virginia was lead author for WABA's Action Folder on BFHI a decade ago. She is a member of WABA's International Advisory Council (1999-2013). A cultural historian of the history of medicine, her MA and PhD theses both examine the influences on mothers' infant feeding practices.

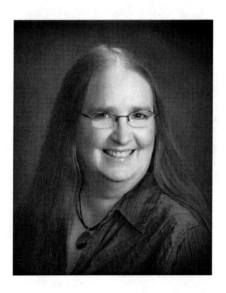

Melissa Clark Vickers. Photo by Don Hayes.

Melissa Clark Vickers, mother of two grown children, is a writer, an International Board Certified Lactation Consultant, and long-time La Leche League Leader. She taught high school biology until the birth of her son Dan in 1983. When her second child, Merrilee, was a year old and not sleeping through the night, in desperation Melissa attended her first LLL meeting in Marietta, Georgia, where she found not only mother support for breastfeeding, but also for a parenting style that resonated with her instincts that said to ignore "conventional wisdom" and instead focus on meeting the needs of her child. She became an LLL Leader in 1990, and resumed her "teaching" career—only this time by helping other mothers discover the satisfaction that comes from parenting from the heart.

Melissa also discovered a love of writing through LLL Leadership, and has written for various international, national, regional, and local publications in and out of LLL. She recently co-authored LLL Founder Marian Tompson's memoir, *Passionate Journey—My Unexpected Life*. In addition, she works extensively with Family Voices, a national organization dedicated to family-centered care and advocacy for families of children with special healthcare needs (www.familyvoices.org). She participated on the American Academy of Pediatrics Infancy Expert Panel for the 2008 revision of *Bright Futures: Guidelines for Health Supervision of Infants, Children, and Adolescents, 3rd Edition.*

Melissa and her husband, Bob, live in rural west Tennessee.

Ordering Information

Hale Publishing, L.P.

1712 N. Forest Street

Amarillo, Texas, USA 79106

8:00 am to 5:00 pm CST

Call » 806.376.9900

Toll free » 800.378.1317

Fax » 806.376.9901

Online Orders

www.ibreastfeeding.com